I would like to dedicate this work to the memory of the late Dr. Johnny D. Ouzts.

Thank you for your friendship and guidance; without it I would not have made it this far.

ACKNOWLEDGEMENTS

My deepest gratitude is extended to Dr. Kuell Hinson for serving as my mentor throughout my program of study. I would also like to thank the remaining members of my graduate committee, Drs. Joe Funderburk, Ken Quesenberry, John Strayer, and David Wofford, for their insight and guidance. This study could not have been completed without the support and aid of the USDA-ARS Soybean Production Research Unit at Stoneville, Mississippi. I want to thank each and every member for their friendship, patience, and support during this educational process. Also, I would like to thank Dr. Clarence Watson and Debbie Boykin for their statistical advice. A special thanks goes to Drs. Edgar E. Hartwig and Thomas C. Kilen for taking a chance on a young kid years ago, and introducing me to the wonderful field of plant breeding.

TABLE OF CONTENTS

LIST OF TABLES

LIST OF FIGURES

Abstract of Dissertation Presented to the Graduate School
of the University of Florida in Partial Fulfillment of the
Requirements for the Degree of
Doctor of Philosophy

INHERITANCE OF RESISTANCE TO THE SOYBEAN LOOPER
IN SOYBEAN

By

Michael Montgomery Kenty

April, 1994

Chairman: Kuell Hinson
Major Department: Agronomy

Phytophagous insects cause millions of dollars of damage to soybean [*Glycine max*

(L.) Merr.] throughout the southern United States. This study was conducted to: (*i*)

evaluate three methods for rating defoliation of soybean by insects and (*ii*) determine the

inheritance of resistance to the soybean looper [*Pseudoplusia includens* Walker] in

soybean. The insect-resistant breeding line D86-3429 was crossed with the cultivar

Braxton in 1988. Additional crosses were made in 1989 and 1990 to provide the

populations necessary to conduct rating methodology and genetic studies in field cages

in 1990 and 1991. The three rating methods evaluated were whole plant visual (WP),

partitioned plant average visual (AV), and measured average leaf area of partitioned plant

(AL). In 1990 the WP and AL were highly correlated (r=0.65, p < 0.001) and in 1991

all correlations (WP vs. AV, WP vs. AL, and AV vs. AL) were significant at p <

0.001. Based on the relative variation of each method, the precision of the three methods was essentially equal and very good, well below the desirable level of 10. These results indicated that relative estimates are suitable for genetic studies. In the inheritance study defoliation was estimated by the WP method in 1990 and the AV method in 1991. The data from the preliminary study in 1990 showed a trend towards quantitative inheritance, therefore the 1991 data were analyzed quantitatively. Mather's scaling test was applied to the data generated from each cage and the results indicated that generation means depend only on additive gene effects. Utilizing Hayman's methodology in terms of the generation means analysis, an epistatic effect was suggested, but the primary effect is assumed to be additive, as was indicated in the scaling test. Estimates of gene numbers indicate that the two parents differed by two genes for resistance to soybean looper. Heritability for resistance was estimated to be 63%, therefore a breeder should be able to make progress by selecting in the F_2 or F_3 populations. The potential exists for increasing resistance to the soybean looper, and possibly other phytophagous insects, by pyramiding genes from new sources of resistance.

CHAPTER 1
INTRODUCTION

Soybean [*Glycine max* (L.) Merrill] is a major world crop. Total world hectares planted increased from 47.1 million in 1977-78 to 57.7 million in 1989-90 (2,3). This 22.5% increase was due primarily to demand for oil and meal products, and to a small extent the whole bean product (75). In the United States, hectarage rose to a peak of 28.6 million hectares in 1978-79 with a steady decline to 24.0 million hectares in 1989-90. This 16% decrease in soybean hectarage was primarily due to reduced plantings in the southeastern United States (3).

The reduction in hectares planted to soybean in the southeastern United States is attributable to the low market value of soybean. Another reason for the reduction is the inability of farmers, in general, to effectively produce a profitable crop in the presence of yield-reducing factors. These factors include fungal diseases, viral diseases, bacterial diseases, nematodes, insects, and drought. In 1982, Mississippi suffered an estimated $50 million loss in revenue from insects alone, of which $40 million could be attributed solely to the soybean looper, *Pseudoplusia includens* Walker (15). Similar losses also occurred in states neighboring Mississippi as a result of insect infestations (15,16). Pest problems which can be costly to control, and a 10-year (1981-1990) average price of $6.19 per bu (3), make it increasingly difficult for a grower to produce a profitable crop.

Several techniques are available for control of diseases, nematodes, and insects in soybean. Metcalf and Luckmann (50) categorized these techniques into seven major methods: cultural, mechanical, physical, biological, chemical, genetic, and regulatory. All methods of control have merit and should be utilized in integrated pest management programs (14,20,58,50). Although economics is the major limiting factor in achieving control of any pest of soybean, human safety and environmental impact must be considered when choosing an approach to control a particular pest. Before making a decision on what approach to take, a grower should answer the questions: 'Will the end results justify the cost of control?' and 'Is the control measure safe?'.

The soybean looper has become increasingly resistant to available insecticides (10,18,48,58,60). For control of the soybean looper and other insect pests, a biological approach should yield the best results. There are two biological approaches to insect control: host plant resistance and the use of biocontrol agents (14,58). The latter involves the identification and exploitation of natural enemies and pathogens. This method of control usually is limited to a specific insect pest rather than the broad spectrum of insects that damage soybean. As with conventional insecticides, resistance to microbial insecticides has been observed (58).

Host plant resistance offers an effective method of control which is built into the plant. It has relatively long stability, is compatible with other control tactics, is environmentally safe (58), and development and subsequent release of a resistant cultivar is far more socially acceptable (82). Lambert and Kilen (47) found that direct selection for resistance in soybean to one species of insect resulted in the indirect selection for resistance to certain other species. The development of an insect-resistant soybean cultivar takes approximately the same amount of time as is required to develop a new, effective insecticide, which can be as short as 10 to 12 years or as long as 20 years. The insect-resistant cultivars 'Lamar' (28) and 'Crockett' (5) each took approximately 20 years to develop.

Initially, Van Duyn et al. (83) identified the three plant introductions PI 171451, PI 227687, and PI 229358 from the USDA germplasm collection as having the highest level of resistance to the Mexican bean beetle (*Epilachna varivestis* Mulsant). Schillinger (69) identified additional sources of resistance to specific insects and described the mechanism of resistance that each exhibits. Hatchett et al. (30) determined that breeding lines identified as possessing resistance to multiple species of insects could serve as basic germplasm for development of cultivars resistant to insects. To date, two soybean cultivars and two soybean germplasm lines with resistance to insects have been registered with the Crop Science Society of America (5,11,28,29).

Although there has been success in developing insect-resistant germplasm lines and cultivars, there has been very little research conducted on the inheritance of insect resistance in soybean (37,54,72). Of the three inheritance studies, two (54,72) were conducted on the resistance to Mexican bean beetle and one (37) on the resistance to the velvetbean caterpillar (*Anticarsia gemmatalis* Hubner). Since the soybean looper is a major pest to soybean in the southeastern United States and is difficult to control with insecticides, the inheritance of resistance to the soybean looper would aid breeders in the development of resistant cultivars.

The objectives of this study were: (*i*) to evaluate three methods for rating defoliation of soybean by soybean looper and (*ii*) to determine the inheritance of resistance in soybean to the soybean looper.

CHAPTER 2
LITERATURE REVIEW

Although undocumented, plants that are resistant to insects have survived and propagated based on the processes of adaptation and natural selection. These 'survivors' were in turn selected by farmers to plant future crops (74). This practice of selection by primitive farmers could be considered the beginning of the development of insect-resistant cultivars.

According to Kogan (38), Pedigo (58), and Smith (74), in their brief histories of insect-resistant plants, the first development and subsequent cultivation of insect-resistant cultivars occurred in the late eighteenth and early nineteenth centuries. In 1792, J.N. Havens identified the wheat (*Triticum aestivium* L. em. Thell.) cultivar 'Underhill' as being resistant to the Hessian fly *(Mayetiola destructor* Say). In the 1830's, G. Lindley recommended the cultivation of apple (*Malus pumila* Miller) cultivars resistant to the woolly apple aphid (*Eriosoma lanigerum* Hausman). In the mid-nineteenth century, the French wine industry was saved by grafting the highly susceptible scions of the French varieties to the rootstocks of American grapes (*Vitis* L. spp.), which were resistant to the grape phylloxera (*Phylloxera vittifolae* Fitch).

In the United States, R.H. Painter is considered to be the founder and pioneer of the modern era of research on insect-resistant plants (58,74). In his book, *Insect*

Resistance in Crop Plants, which was the first book written on the topic, he described mechanisms of resistance in plants and factors that affect them. Based on field observations, he separated the mechanisms of resistance in plants into three distinct, but interactive classes: nonpreference, later known as antixenosis (38), (for oviposition, food, or shelter), antibiosis (adverse effect on the biology of the insect), and tolerance (ability to withstand, repair, or recover from infestation) (57). Developing a cultivar that exhibits a high level of all three mechanisms of resistance would be optimum. This is seldom feasible, therefore developing cultivars with the antibiosis mechanism of resistance is the most frequent objective of plant breeders. Although nonpreference and antibiosis differ in their mechanisms of resistance, both involve the interaction of the biology of the plant with the biology of the insect (58,74). There is often an overlapping of the nonpreference and antibiosis classes which makes it difficult to determine the exact mechanism of resistance exhibited in a plant to a particular species of insect (74).

Although it is advantageous if a breeder knows which mechanism of resistance is being expressed, knowledge of the mechanism is not essential to make advances in the development of resistant germplasm. In fact, resistant cultivars and germplasm have been developed for years with little concern for the underlying mechanism of resistance. It has only been in the past two decades that mechanisms of resistance have been identified in crop plants (39).

In soybean, Van Duyn et al. (83) identified three genotypes (PI 171451, PI 227687, and PI 229358) from the USDA germplasm collection of maturity groups VII and VIII as resistant to the Mexican bean beetle. These three PI's have been used extensively as sources of resistant germplasm and as standard checks in screening additional germplasm for resistance. At the World Soybean Research Conference in 1975, Schillinger (69) reported additional sources of resistance to the Mexican bean beetle. Gary et al. (22) screened 1108 lines from maturity groups VI, VII, VIII, and IX of the USDA germplasm collection against velvetbean caterpillar initially, and subsequently velvetbean caterpillar, soybean looper, corn earworm (*Heliothis zea* Boddie), tobacco budworm (*H. virescens* Fabricius), and beet armyworm (*Spodoptera exigua* Hubner). Based on the results of the screenings against these five species, PI 209837 and FC 31592 were identified as having levels of resistance that would be suitable for developing resistant cultivars. The germplasm collection of 473 PI's of wild soybean, *Glycine soja* Sieb. & Zucc., was screened against soybean looper, velvetbean caterpillar, beet armyworm, and corn earworm to identify additional sources of resistance equal to, or greater than, PI's 229358 and 171451. McKenna et al. (52) identified three lines (PI's 464935-1, 366119, and 407301) from this study as having less defoliation than the two standards, thus suggesting that there are additional genes for insect resistance. In 1988, Kraemer et al. (42) identified several accessions of the USDA germplasm collection as being resistant to the Mexican bean beetle. They were from maturity groups VI (FC 31665, and PI's 379621, 416925, and 416937) and VIII (PI's 417061 and 417136).

Upon identification of a genotype that is resistant to a certain insect species, the genotype usually is screened against other insect species. Resistance to more than one species will enhance its usefulness in a breeding program. Hatchett et al. (30) conducted a study utilizing breeding lines that derive their insect resistance from PI 229358 to determine if selection for resistance to one or two insect species would result in the indirect selection for resistance to other troublesome species. They found that no single insect species could be utilized to select for resistance to multiple species of insects among adapted genotypes. In a similar study, Lambert and Kilen (47) determined that when PI 229358 was used as the donor parent, direct selection for resistance to one insect species resulted in indirect selection for resistance to other foliar-feeding species.

Research to develop soybean genotypes resistant to insects is usually conducted with species that are indigenous to a particular area (19,25,35,44,54,64,80,83). Lambert and Kilen (45) evaluated PI 229358, PI 227687, and PI 171451 against five insect species to determine their relative levels of resistance. Insect species tested were velvetbean caterpillar, soybean looper, corn earworm, tobacco budworm, and beet armyworm. Based upon the responses to these five species, they found that the mechanism for resistance in PI 171451 was nonpreference, whereas that of PI 229358 or PI 227687 was antibiosis. These same three PI's were evaluated against four important soybean defoliating species (beet armyworm, *Porthesia taiwania* Shiraki, *Anomala cupripes* Bates, and *Orgyia* species) to determine their usefulness in developing breeding lines resistant to insects indigenous to Taiwan. No single accessions had a consistently high level of resistance to all of the insect species. PI 227687 demonstrated the highest level of resistance to the most prevalent species, the beet armyworm, and therefore would be suitable to initiate a breeding program (80).

With the sources of resistance to various species of insects identified, researchers have channelled their energy into determining the basis of the mechanism of resistance in certain soybean accessions. Since the mid-1970's, researchers have investigated various constituents of soybean to identify the underlying biochemical compound that confers resistance to insects (9,53,73,81). If an association could be established between a particular compound or class of compounds and resistance, then a new tool could be developed to accelerate the selection process by breeders.

In studies with PI 227687, PI 229358, and two susceptible cultivars, Tester (81) reported that resistant PI's had lower total nitrogen, more soluble carbohydrates, and more total sterols at flowering and pod-fill than susceptible cultivars. Through a series of grafting experiments, Lambert and Kilen (46) verified that constituents contributing to resistance in PI 227687 and PI 229358 were formed in the leaves and translocated throughout the plant. Smith (73) determined that the resistant factors in PI 227687 appeared to be chemical. He also found that resistance to the soybean looper in PI 227687 was an antibiotic effect due to the combined effects of a feeding deterrent and a growth inhibitor. Chiang et al. (9) suggested that resistance to Mexican bean beetle feeding in PI 227687 may be attributed to phenylpropanoid metabolites. In their inorganic nutrient analysis of leaf tissue studies with soybean resistant to the Mexican bean beetle, Mebrahtu et al. (53) found that the content of calcium, phosphorus, and potassium was negatively correlated with pupal weight gain ($r = -0.23^{**}$, $r = -0.26^{**}$, and $r = -0.20^{*}$; $p < 0.01$ and $p < 0.05$, respectively).

In 1986, Kogan (39) published a treatise on the role of biochemicals in plant resistance to insects. He examined the defensive patterns of three families: Solanaceae, Cruciferae, and Leguminosae (specifically the common bean and soybean) and published, as quoted below, a summation of all previous research findings that elucidated the chemical bases of resistance in PI 171451, PI 227687, and PI 229358.

1. Foliar total nitrogen, soluble carbohydrates, organic acids and sterols of both resistant and susceptible soybean vary with stage of growth (Tester, 1977; Grunwald and Kogan, 1981).

2. Total nitrogen was generally lower and, at the end of the season, soluble carbohydrates and sterols were higher in the resistant lines; organic acids fluctuated without correlation with resistance (Testor, 1977).

3. Sterol profiles were similar in both susceptible and resistant lines, both in early and in late maturing soybeans (Grunwald and Kogan, 1981).

4. Pinitol is a dominant cyclitol in soybean and it represents an average of 60% of the total 80%-ethanol-soluble carbohydrate fraction of soybean (Phillips et al., 1982).

5. Pinitol was found in large amounts in PI 229358, and in smaller concentrations in the susceptible cultivar 'Davis' (@ 1% dry weight). Added to artificial media at 0.8%, pinitol reduced weight gain by corn earworm larvae by about 63%. These findings suggest that pinitol is an antibiotic factor in soybean but with no apparent antixenotic property (Dreyer et al., 1979). As the reported results could not be replicated elsewhere, this claim has been recently disputed (Gardner et al., 1984).

6. Systematic fractionation of PI's 227687 (Smith and Fischer, 1983) and 229358 (Binder and Waiss, 1984) yielded fractions with intermediate and with polar solvents that caused slower developmental rates and high mortality in soybean looper [*Pseudoplusia includens* (Walker)] and *Heliothis zea* Boddie, respectively.

7. Seven phenolic acids were detected in PI 171451 and in cv. 'Forrest'; gallic, protocatechuic, p-hydroxybenzoic, vanillic, caffeic, p-coumaric, and ferulic. The potentially antibiotic caffeic and ferulic acids occurred at higher concentrations in the resistant PI than in the susceptible cultivar. In both types of plants, concentrations were higher in injured than in uninjured tissue (Hardin, 1979).

8. Isoflavonoid phytoalexins in soybean cotyledons are potent feeding deterrents for the Mexican bean beetle (Hart et al., 1983). These phytoalexins are biochemically related to the phenolics mentioned above, through the shikimic pathway. (39, p.516-518).

Although a great deal of knowledge has been gained, there still remain many unanswered questions as to what components comprise the various mechanisms of resistance.

A moderate amount of research has been conducted in the area of resistance in soybean to insects, and much progress has been made in cultivar development. However, there has been very little information published on the inheritance of resistance to insects in soybean. In their work with the Mexican bean beetle, Sisson et al. (72) hypothesized that resistance was inherited quantitatively and that the number of major genes involved was small, perhaps two or three major genes. In further studies with the Mexican bean beetle, Mebrahtu et al. (54) concluded that resistance appeared to be primarily an expression of additive genetic variance. Kilen et al. (36), in their studies with the soybean looper, suggested that susceptibility was partially dominant with a few major genes conditioning resistance. In their studies with PI 171451, PI 227687, and PI 229358, and the F_1 plants derived from intercrosses among the three PI's, Lambert and Kilen (45) suggested that genetic resistance in PI 171451 differed from that operating in the other two lines. This was further supported by their work with the PI's and the F_3

lines derived from the intercrosses among the PI's. They hypothesized that each PI contained a resistance gene that differed from those of the other lines. To design a better breeding program to develop cultivars resistant to the soybean looper utilizing breeding lines that derive their insect resistance from PI 229358, it would be advantageous if the mode of inheritance of this trait were known.

CHAPTER 3
EVALUATION OF RATING METHODS

Introduction

Throughout the past 25 years there have been advances in the identification and development of soybean breeding lines resistant to phytophagous insects, especially Lepidopterous species and the Mexican bean beetle (5,11,22,28,29,30,42,52,79,83). Despite these advances, little effort has been devoted to improving the methods of evaluating the amount of feeding injury of insects. Most researchers utilize a rating system that estimates the level of resistance among cultivars, but little or no effort has been made to determine whether or not the rating scales used were truly reflecting the defoliation caused by insects. Hence, the objective of this study was to evaluate the effectiveness of the widely used visual, or relative, assessment of insect defoliation as compared to a quantitative, or absolute, assessment.

Literature Review

Plant pathologists have faced problems in the assessment of disease which is dependent upon the causal organism and the host plant species. Many different methods of disease assessment are available to plant pathologists (7). Shokes et al. (71) tested the reliability of disease assessment procedures with late leafspot [*Cercosporidium personatum* (Berk. and Curt.) Deighton] in peanut (*Arachis hypogaea* L.) and concluded that plant pathologists would benefit if a standard rating system for foliar diseases of peanut could be adopted as has been done in other crops. In a special report, Berger (4) stated that a disease assessment procedure should have the following basic requirements: easy to learn, quick and efficient to use, applicable across a broad spectrum of conditions, and be accurate, precise, and reproducible. He concluded that the greater the emphasis placed on the assessment method, the higher the quality of information obtained by the method.

In 1980, Kogan and Turnipseed (41) described the various methods of quantitative and qualitative assessments of defoliation that are currently used by researchers working with phytophagous insects. These methods are: (*i*) photoelectric or electronic (measure actual leaf area), (*ii*) gravimetric (regressing known leaf areas on the corresponding fresh or dry weight of these areas, (*iii*) volumetric (volume displacement cylinder is used to measure biomass), (*iv*) planimetric (mechanical measurement of area), (*v*) geometric (estimates total nondefoliated leaf area so that percent defoliation can be calculated when used in conjunction with a leaf area meter), and (*vi*) visual estimates (provide rapid estimate of defoliation). Although descriptions of the methods were detailed by Kogan and Turnipseed, no statistical comparisons were made among methods.

Some authors (58,78) refer to qualitative assessments as relative estimates and quantitative assessments as absolute estimates. Relative estimates do not translate directly into the amount of defoliation, whereas absolute estimates allow for direct translation into the amount of defoliation caused by phytophagous insects. The major drawback of absolute estimates is that they are usually time consuming and costly to make.

Conversely, relative estimates can be timely and are inexpensive which is why these types of estimates are more widely used by researchers (74).

Funderburk et al. (19) determined that plot size or shape had little effect on the relative rankings of soybean cultivars when measuring resistance to the velvetbean caterpillar in terms of percentage of defoliation based on visual estimates. However, they found that the mean and precision of the estimates were affected by plot size and shape. The objective of this study was to compare two relative methods to one absolute method for assessing defoliation caused by the soybean looper.

Materials and Methods

The three rating methods evaluated in 1990 and 1991 were the whole plant visual rating (WP), the partitioned plant average visual rating (AV), and measured average leaf area of the partitioned plant (AL). WP values were based on a 1-to-10 scale divided into 10% increments with a score of 1 signifying defoliation of 0 to 10% and a score of 10 signifying defoliation of 91 to 100%. Although other scales, such as a logarithmic scale (33), may be better at estimating defoliation, the 1-to-10 scale was chosen since it is most commonly used by participants in the Regional Host Plant Resistance Test which is sponsored annually by the Southern Regional Information Exchange Group (SRIEG - 32). With the AV and AL methods, the canopies were visually partitioned into three sections (top, middle, bottom) enabling a more detailed assessment of soybean looper defoliation on each plant. The partitioning of the plants was based on a procedure that was developed by Plaut and Berger (59) that was cited by Shokes et al. (71). For AV estimates, each section of the plant was scored using the same scale as the WP with the three scores averaged to obtain the AV.

In 1990, a LI-COR LI-3000 (Li-Cor, Inc., Lincoln, NE 68504) portable leaf area meter was used to measure the middle leaflet of a representative trifoliate from each of the sections and the three measurements were averaged to obtain the AL. In 1990 the AL method only allowed an indirect comparison to the other two methods, therefore the AL was modified in 1991 to permit a direct comparison with AV and WP. In the 1991 AL method, a representative trifoliolate leaf from each section of the partitioned plant was removed and taken into a laboratory to determine the area of each sample. The portable leaf area meter was used to determine the remaining portion of each defoliated leaflet (DEF) of each trifoliolate. Following the procedure described by Kogan and Turnipseed (41), each leaflet of the trifoliolates was then placed on a photocopy machine and a copy was made. Examples of leaflet photocopies are shown in Figure 1. These silhouettes were then cut out to represent the trifoliolates in a nondefoliated state and the area (NONDEF) for each was determined as mentioned above. The two values obtained for each trifoliolate were used in the following formula to determine the percent defoliation (% def): (NONDEF - DEF)/NONDEF * 100 = % def. The percent defoliation for each of the three trifoliolates from each plant was then converted to the same 1-to-10 scale used by the other two methods and the values averaged, allowing direct comparisons to be made among the three methods.

The plants used in the evaluation of the three methods were part of an inheritance study that was conducted in field cages (43) in 1990 and 1991 at the Mississippi State

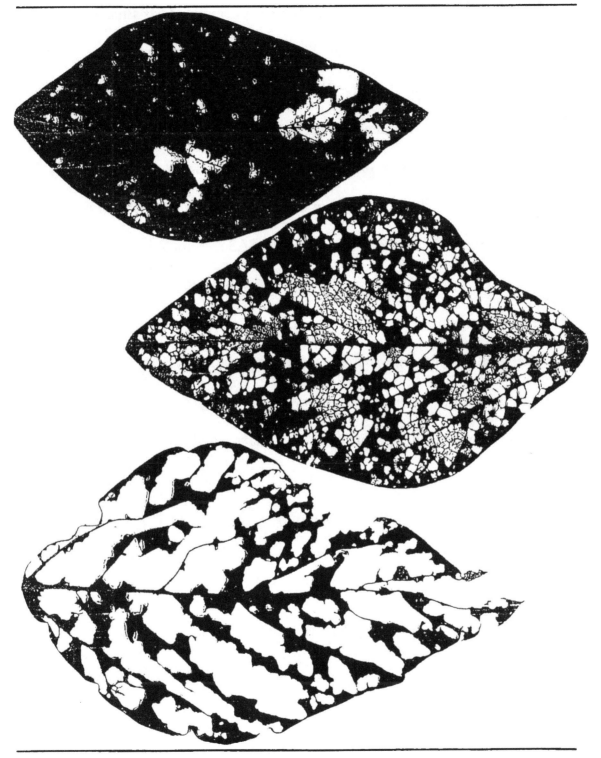

Figure 1. Examples of photocopied leaflets used in determining the % defoliation in the AV (leaf area of partitioned plant) method.

University Delta Research and Extension Center, Stoneville, Mississippi. In the first year of the study, seed were planted on 25 May 1990. In 1991, seed were planted on 25 May and 29 May in cage 1, and on 31 May in cage 2. Rainfall on 25 May prevented completion of planting on the same day in cage 1.

To compare methods in 1990, ten soybean plants were chosen randomly from each of 20 backcross families for a total of 200 plants. Fifty plants in each of two cages were randomly chosen using PROC PLAN of PC-SAS (68) for use in the evaluation of the three methods in 1991. These plants were chosen prior to release of soybean looper moths in both years.

The 4000 three-day-old soybean looper moths were released on 25 June 1990 when plants were at the V5 to V6 stage of plant growth (17). Larvae from hatched eggs were allowed to feed freely for approximately 12 days, at which time 'Centennial' (27), the susceptible check, was estimated to have a rating of nine according to the WP method. The area within the cage was then sprayed with methomyl [S-methyl-N-((methyl carbamoyl) oxy)-thioacetimidate] at 0.5 kg ha^{-1} to kill the larvae. This allowed defoliation ratings to be made without further feeding. The day following spraying, each plant was rated by all three methods.

Approximately 4000 three-day-old soybean looper moths were released into each cage on 8 July 1991. At the time of release, plants in cage 1 were V7 to V8 and in cage 2 they were V6 to V7. The larvae from the hatched eggs were allowed to feed freely until the susceptible check, Centennial, received a rating of ten by the WP method, 16 days after release of the moths. To cease feeding at this stage of plant growth, R1 to R2 in cage 1 and beginning R1 in cage 2, the plants in both cages were sprayed with methomyl at 0.5 kg ha^{-1} to kill the larvae. The following day each of the 100 plants was rated using the WP and AV methods and samples were collected for the AL.

Data derived from each rating method for the 200 plants in 1990 and the 100 plants in 1991 were subjected to analytical procedures in PC-SAS (68). A correlation analysis was run to determine the correlation coefficient (r) between WP and AL, AV and WP, and AL and WP rating methods each year. A paired difference comparison (76) was made between WP and AV methods in 1990 and between WP and AL, WP and AV, and AL and AV methods in 1991. McNemar's test for concordance (77) was used to test for significant changes between WP and AL in 1990 and between WP and AL, WP and AV, and AL and AV methods in 1991. This analysis was conducted to determine if the methods differed in their estimates of defoliation. Precision, known as the relative variation (RV), of the two relative methods for both years and the absolute method in 1991 were calculated for each as follows:

$$RV = (SE/\bar{x})100$$

where SE is the standard error of the mean and $\bar{x}$ is the mean. This relationship, described by Ruesink (66) and Pedigo (58), is considered useful in estimating precision of a sampling method by entomologists.

Results and Discussion

The 1990 scores for each of the three rating methods by plant are presented in Appendix A. Scores for AV and WP were based on a 1-to-10 scale, with lower numbers indicating less defoliation. The measurements for AL in 1990 are presented as cm^2 of remaining tissue. Individual plant data for each of the three methods in 1991 are presented in Appendix B. Unlike 1990, 1991 data for all three methods were based on a 1-to-10 scale. Means and standard deviations for both years are also reported in Appendices A and B.

Frequency distributions of the 1990 WP and AV rating methods are shown in Figure 2. The AL method was omitted from this graph because it measured the remaining undefoliated tissue in cm^2, whereas the AV and WP methods were used to estimate percent defoliation on a 1-to-10 scale. Frequency distributions of the AV and WP methods suggest that either the evaluator underestimated defoliation by the WP method or overestimated defoliation by the AV method. Without an absolute estimate of defoliation, no substantial conclusion can be made as to the reliability of AV or WP to accurately assess defoliation.

The 1991 frequency distributions of all three methods for both cages combined are presented in Figure 3. Due to the modifications in the AL method, it was possible to make direct comparisons between AL and the visual rating methods. The evaluator overestimated defoliation to obtain too few plants below 30% or <4 in the 1-to-10 scale when using either relative method, WP or AV, as compared to AL, the absolute method. Also, the evaluator had a tendency to overestimate the amount of defoliation over 50% or >5 in the 1-to-10 scale when using either relative method as compared to AL. Only in classes 4, 5, and 6 was the evaluator's estimate of defoliation with the WP and AV methods similar to that of the AL. The problem of overestimating might be avoided in

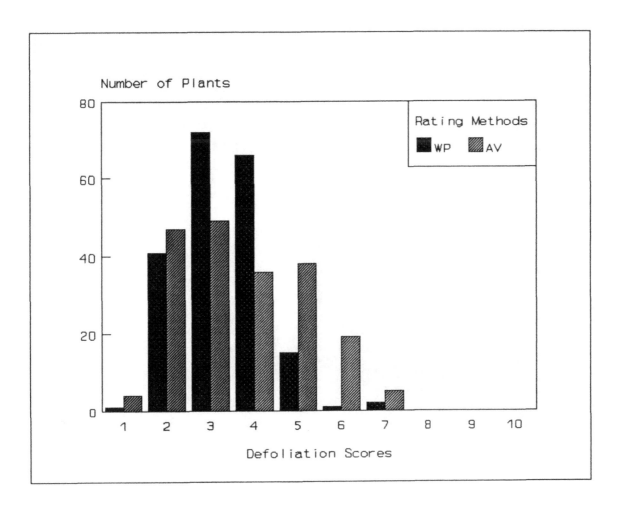

Figure 2. 1990 frequency distribution of defoliation estimates by the whole plant and partitioned plant average visual rating methods. Defoliation scores based on 1-to-10 scale where 1 = 0 to 10% defoliation, 2 = 11 to 20%, 3 = 21 to 30%, 4 = 31 to 40%, 5 = 41 to 50%, 6 = 51 to 60%, 7 = 61 to 70%, 8 = 71 to 80%, 9 = 81 to 90%, 10 = 91 to 100%.

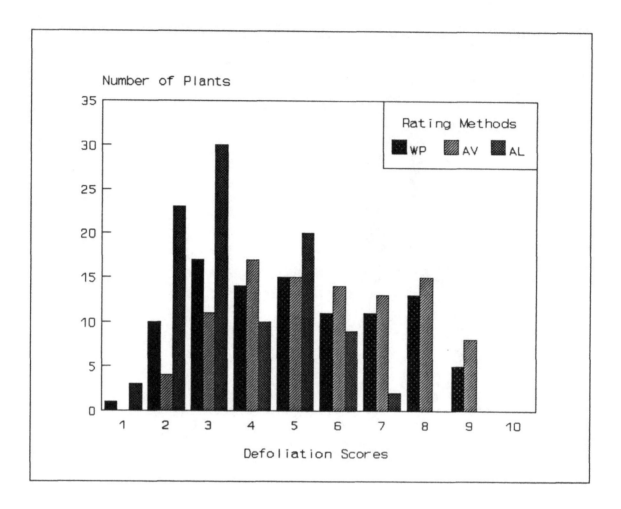

Figure 3. 1991 frequency distribution of defoliation estimates by the whole plant, partitioned plant average visual, and measured average leaf area of the partitioned plant rating methods. Defoliation scores based on 1-to-10 scale where 1 = 0 to 10% defoliation, 2 = 11 to 20%, 3 = 21 to 30%, 4 = 31 to 40%, 5 = 41 to 50%, 6 = 51 to 60%, 7 = 61 to 70%, 8 = 71 to 80%, 9 = 81 to 90%, 10 = 91 to 100%.

the future if a logarithmic rating scale, such as the Horsefall-Barratt scale to assess disease (33), were used to estimate defoliation. A logarithmic scale may have advantages for assessment of defoliation because the visual acuity of the human eye is more adapted to the identification of small differences at each end of the scale.

The plant scores of the AV and the WP rating methods in 1990 were highly correlated ($r = 0.65$, $p < 0.001$). AL measurements were in cm^2 of nondefoliated leaf area remaining, therefore not a measure of defoliation. As there was no absolute measure of defoliation, it was not possible to make further comparisons with AV and WP.

In 1991, the scores for cage 1 from the AV and WP methods were significantly correlated with the AL method ($r = 0.86$, $p < 0.001$; and $r = 0.88$, $p < 0.001$, respectively). The AV and WP methods correlated well with each other ($r = 0.88$, $p < 0.001$). By squaring each of the correlation coefficients (r), both the WP vs. AV and WP vs. AL relationships had r^2 values of 0.77 meaning 77% of the variance in one rating method can be explained by the variation in the other. The AV vs. AL correlation had a r^2 value of 0.74, indicating that 74% of the variance of the AV method can be explained by the variation in the AL method (or vice versa).

Although the results from ratings on plants in cage 2 were similar, correlations were not as high as those in cage 1. Scores from the AV and WP methods were significantly correlated with the AL method ($r = 0.75$, $p < 0.001$; and $r = 0.67$, $p < 0.001$, respectively). The AV and WP methods were significantly correlated ($r = 0.74$, $p < 0.001$) with each other. Calculated r^2 values were: WP vs. AV $r^2 = 0.55$, WP vs.

AL $r^2 = 0.49$, and AV vs. AL $r^2 = 0.56$. These values are lower than those found with the cage 1 data. Differences may be attributed to differences in the plant growth at the time of rating or to evaluator error. The cage 2 ratings were made in the rain which hindered the evaluator's ability to accurately estimate defoliation. It was considered more prudent to make ratings in the rain than to attempt to disregard the ensuing regrowth which was increasing rapidly during a prolonged rainy period.

When data for both cages were pooled for analysis, scores for the AV and WP methods were significantly correlated with the AL method ($r = 0.79$, $p < 0.001$; and $r = 0.78$, $p < 0.001$, respectively). The AV and WP methods correlated well with each other ($r = 0.80$, $p < 0.001$) as in the cages treated separately. The following r^2 values were obtained: WP vs. AV $r^2 = 0.64$, WP vs. AL $r^2 = 0.60$, and AV vs. AL $r^2 = 0.62$ thus approximately 62% ($\pm$ 2%) of the variation in one rating method could be attributed to the variation in the other rating method.

In a similar study, a relative method and an absolute method were compared using their estimates of defoliation of field plots infested primarily (90% of total insect population) with the velvetbean caterpillar (G.R. Bowers, 1992, personal communication). A 1-to-9 scale, with 1 signifying the least damage, was used as the relative method. The absolute method followed a procedure described by Kogan and Kuhlman (40) in which 20 leaflets each from the top, middle, and bottom thirds of plants (for a total of 60) were sampled from plants located in the center two rows of a four-row plot. These were then compared to diagrams of defoliated leaves to determine the defoliation estimate of each sample. The two methods were significantly correlated, r

$= 0.62, p < 0.001$. Bower's correlation coefficients are somewhat similar to the pooled correlation coefficients between the relative and absolute methods in this 1991 cage experiment.

Correlations from the 1991 experiment, whether examined individually by cage or combined, were all significant at $p < 0.001$. The magnitude of the r^2 values indicate that the evaluator obtained similar relative rankings of defoliation regardless the method used. Although the correlations between the AL method and the WP and AV methods were highly significant, it was not possible to determine if the evaluator estimated the same amount of defoliation with the WP and AV methods (relative methods) as with the AL method (the absolute method). To compare the accuracy of the evaluator using the two relative methods and the absolute method, additional analyses were undertaken.

With the PROC MEANS procedure of PC-SAS, a paired difference comparison was made between the WP and AV methods in 1990. A t-test was performed to test the equality of the two methods based on the differences between the two methods for each plant in the study. The mean difference of -0.36 between the WP and AV methods was highly significant, $p < 0.001$, meaning the WP method yielded lower average percent defoliation than the AV method. However, without some measure of the actual or absolute defoliation across the plants, there was no way to determine if the evaluator could obtain an accurate assessment of the true defoliation of a plant with either method.

A paired difference comparison was also made among the three rating methods in 1991. The WP and AV methods had a mean difference of -0.55, $p < 0.001$, which was somewhat similar in magnitude to the mean difference calculated in the 1990 study.

The mean differences $\pm$ standard deviation involving the AL method were 1.48 $\pm$ 0.14 for WP - AL and 2.03 $\pm$ 0.12 for AV - AL, respectively. Both differences were significant at the $p < 0.001$ level. Although the evaluator estimated a higher average percent defoliation with both relative methods than with the absolute method, the estimate obtained with the WP method was numerically more similar to the measured defoliation obtained with the AL method.

With the relative methods, WP and AV, the evaluator estimated somewhat similar amounts of defoliation across all plants when compared with each other, even though the difference between the two methods was highly significant. However, in comparisons with an absolute method, AL, it becomes apparent that the evaluator's estimates of defoliation with the WP method were closer to the actual than were the estimates of the AV method. Although the AL method is accepted as the absolute measure of defoliation for each plant, there is some evidence that it underestimated defoliation. Necrotic leaf tissue due to insect injury was present. The leaf area meter could not distinguish viable leaf tissue from necrotic tissue. The amount of necrotic tissue was not enough to increase AL values to the level of WP value, however the best absolute estimate of defoliation would have been to sample the entire plant (destructive sampling) and follow the protocol of the AL method after cutting out necrotic tissue. In the 1991 experiment, provisions were not made for destructive sampling; therefore it was not practiced.

McNemar's test for concordance was used to determine if the categorization of plants having less than or equal to 50% defoliation and of plants having greater than 50% defoliation differed with the WP and AV methods. In 1990, 36 of the 198 of the plants were classified with the WP method as having at most 50% defoliation while with the AV method these same plants were rated as having greater than 50% defoliation (Table 1). This percentage (18%) of plants was significantly different from zero, $X^2 = 34.03$, $p < 0.001$, supporting the earlier contention (Figure 2) that either the WP method underestimated defoliation or the AV method overestimated defoliation. Without the absolute method for reference it was not possible to determine which method was more accurate.

All three methods were compared in 1991 to determine whether significant differences among the methods existed. The results from McNemar's test for concordance of the 1991 data are shown in Table 1. The two relative methods were significantly different ($X^2 = 11.25$, $p < 0.001$) with 20 of the 97 plants being classified differently by WP than AV. The relative methods were both significantly different from the absolute method (WP vs. AL $X^2 = 22.04$, $p < 0.001$; and AV vs. AL $X^2 = 38.03$, $p < 0.001$) in the estimate of defoliation on a plant-by-plant basis. With both relative methods, the evaluator had a tendency to overestimate defoliation as compared to the absolute method. With the AV method 40 of 97 plants were classified as $> 50\%$ defoliated while AL classified these same plants as $\leq 50\%$, whereas with the WP method only 24 of 97 plants were classified $> 50\%$ as compared to the AL method classifying them as $\leq 50\%$. This indicates that the evaluator was able to estimate defoliation closer to the absolute method with the WP method as was seen in the paired difference comparison.

Table 1. McNemar test for significant differences between the WP (whole plant visual) and AV (partitioned plant visual) methods in 1990; and between the WP and AV, WP and AL (leaf area of the partitioned plant), and AV and AL methods in 1991.

1990

AV	WP 1 - 5†	WP > 5†	Totals	X^2
1 - 5	159	0	159	
> 5	36	3	39	
Totals	195	3	198	34.03***

1991

AV	WP 1 - 5	WP > 5		
1 - 5	39	2	41	
> 5	18	38	56	
Totals	57	40	97	11.25***

AL	WP 1 - 5	WP > 5		
1 - 5	57	24	81	
> 5	0	16	16	
Totals	57	40	97	22.04***

AL	AV 1 - 5	AV > 5		
1 - 5	41	40	81	
> 5	0	16	16	
Totals	41	56	97	38.03***

*** Significant at the 0.001 level of probability.

† Defoliation ratings based on a 1-to-10 scale where 1 = 0 to 10% defoliation, 2 = 11 to 20%, 3 = 21 to 30%, 4 = 31 to 40%, 5 = 41 to 50%, 6 = 51 to 60%, 7 = 61 to 70%, 8 = 71 to 80%, 9 = 81 to 90%, 10 = 91 to 100%.

RV values for 1990 were 2.11 and 2.77 for WP and AV, respectively. According to Pedigo (58), RV values less than 10 are desirable in research, but the closer the value is to zero the more precise the method is at making estimates. Although the WP method was numerically better than the AV method, the precision of both methods was essentially equal and very good.

The RV values for each of the methods in 1991 were as follows: WP = 4.26, AV = 3.49, and AL = 4.09. Based on the RV values, the AV method was numerically better than either WP or AL. The AL method was expected to be the most precise since it was the absolute measure of defoliation. However in this study, these values were essentially equal and close to zero, thus the evaluator was fairly precise in making estimates of defoliation with all three methods.

Summary and Conclusions

The objective of this study was to evaluate the effectiveness of the widely used visual, or relative, assessment of insect defoliation as compared to a quantitative, or absolute, assessment. In 1990 no absolute method comparisons were possible, however the WP and AV methods were highly correlated ($r = 0.65$, $p < 0.001$). The evaluator estimated a slightly lower amount of defoliation on the average with the WP method than with the AV. The relative variation of these two relative methods were both less than 3.0 which according to Pedigo (58) is very desirable. Without an adequate absolute method no determination could be made as to which relative method best reflected the actual defoliation.

Adjustments in the method of calculating percent defoliation by the AL method for 1991 allowed for direct evaluations of the two relative methods. All correlations (WP vs. AV, WP vs. AL, and AV vs. AL) were significant at the $p < 0.001$ level, whether the cage data were treated separately or pooled. The two relative estimates of defoliation were significantly correlated with the absolute estimate of defoliation. These results are similar to the findings of a another relative versus an absolute estimation of defoliation conducted in 1985 by G.R. Bowers (G.R. Bowers, 1992, personal communication).

Paired comparisons were made among the methods to test the equality of the methods to rate defoliation. In 1991, the estimates of defoliation by all three methods were significantly different. These findings were validated by McNemar's test for concordance. The WP defoliation estimates were more similar to the AL results, than the AV ratings were to AL.

Based on the RV's of each method, the precision of the AV and WP methods was essentially equal in 1990. Similar results were obtained in 1991 with the AV, WP, and AL methods. In both years the precision of the methods was essentially equal and well below the value of 10 that Pedigo (58) states as being desirable. These results indicate that either relative method is suitable for estimating defoliation.

The results of these studies demonstrate that relative estimates of defoliation can be used effectively in genetic studies or routine screenings of advanced breeding lines. Since the two relative methods yielded similar results, it would be advantageous to use the most economical method.

CHAPTER 4
INHERITANCE OF RESISTANCE
TO SOYBEAN LOOPER IN SOYBEAN

Introduction

During the past three decades great strides have been made in the identification and development of insect-resistant breeding lines of soybean (22,30,42,52,79,83). This research has led to the release of several germplasm lines and cultivars (5,11,28,29) that are resistant to phytophagous insects. Although advances have been made, very little information has been published on the inheritance of resistance to foliar-feeding insects.

Sisson et al. (72) reported that resistance to the Mexican bean beetle was quantitatively inherited with two or three major genes involved. In other inheritance studies, Mebrahtu et al. (54) concluded that resistance to the Mexican bean beetle was primarily an expression of additive genetic variance. Kilen et al. (36) suggested that susceptibility to the soybean looper was partially dominant and a few major genes conditioned resistance. Based on their work with PI 171451, PI 227687, and PI 229358 and the F_1 progeny derived from the intercrosses among the three PI's, Lambert and Kilen (45) suggested that the genetic basis for insect resistance in PI 171451 differed from that in the other two PI's. This was further supported by their work with the three PI's and the F_3 lines derived from intercrosses among the three PI's (37). They hypothesized that each PI contained a distinct resistance gene.

31

To facilitate the design of breeding programs to develop cultivars resistant to the soybean looper, it would be beneficial to understand more completely the mode of inheritance of this trait. Therefore, the objective of this study was to determine the mode of inheritance of resistance to the soybean looper in genotypes derived from crosses involving PI 229358.

Materials and Methods

All aspects of this experiment were conducted at the Mississippi State University, Delta Research and Extension Center at Stoneville, MS on a Bosket fine sandy loam (Mollic Hapludalfs).

1988

To study the inheritance of resistance to soybean looper in soybean, the breeding line D86-3429 was crossed with the cultivar Braxton (32). D86-3429 has white flowers (*w1*), gray pubescence (*t*), sensitivity to metribuzin [4-amino-6-(1,1-dimethylethyl)-3-(methylthio)-1,2,4-triazin-5,(4H)-one] (*hm*), resistance to Phytophthora rot (induced by *Phytophthora megasperma* Drechs. f. sp. *glycinea* T. Kuan & D.C. Erwin) (*Rps1-c*), and resistance to soybean looper. The donor of insect resistance was the germplasm line D75-10169 (29), which derived its resistance from PI 229358 (83). The male parent, Braxton, has purple flowers (*W1*), tawny pubescence (*T*), tolerance to metribuzin (*Hm*), susceptibility to Phytophthora rot (*rps*), and susceptibility to soybean looper. Both parents were of maturity group VII. Hand pollinations (1,60) made in the field produced seven seeds of the cross D86-3429 × Braxton.

<u>1989</u>

The seven F_1 seeds produced in 1988 were space-planted 30.5 cm apart in 91.5-cm rows in the F_1 nursery. Several rows of each parent, D86-3429 and Braxton, were planted at a rate of 14 seeds per meter for crossing purposes. Four F_1 plants emerged and these plants were used as the pollen parents for two backcrosses, D86-3429 $\times$ F_1(D86-3429 $\times$ Braxton) (BC_1) and Braxton $\times$ F_1(D86-3429 $\times$ Braxton) (BC_2). The original cross, D86-3429 $\times$ Braxton, and its reciprocal were also made to provide additional F_1 seed for the following year. Approximately 60 hand pollinations were made for the two backcrosses and the two crosses with the expectation that an adequate number of seed would be produced. The two backcrosses, BC_1 and BC_2, produced fourteen and six seed, respectively. At maturity, the seed from the four F_1 plants were harvested to provide F_2 seed for use in 1990. In addition, seed from both parents were harvested for use in 1990. Seven seeds were produced from the cross D86-3429 $\times$ Braxton and five seeds were produced from the reciprocal cross. The seed of the backcrosses, BC_1 and BC_2, were scarified, treated with metalaxyl [<u>N</u>-(2,6-dimethylphenyl)-<u>N</u>-(methoxyacetyl)alanine methyl ester] to optimize rapid emergence of healthy plants, and planted one seed per pot in 15 L pots filled with soil treated with *Bradyrhizobium japonicum* inoculum in the greenhouse during the winter of 1989-90. Plants were allowed to self-pollinate, thus providing seed of the BS_1 (the selfed generation of BC_1) and BS_2 (the selfed generation of BC_2) generations. At maturity the plants were harvested and threshed with an ALMACO (Allen Machine Co., Nevada, IA 50201) single-plant thresher.

The inheritance study was conducted in a screened field cage 2.4 m high $\times$ 19.2 m wide $\times$ 32.0 m long (43). A schematic of the field cage design is shown in Figure 4. In mid-April the soil was disked twice in opposite directions with a disk harrow. On 23 May the soil was tilled with a spring-tooth harrow to smooth the surface. This was followed with a preplant-incorporated herbicide treatment of clomazone 2-(2-chlorophenyl) methyl-4,4-dimethyl-3-isooxazolidinone and trifluralin [2,6-dinitro-N,N-dipropyl-4-(trifluoromethyl)benzenamine] at 1.12 kg ha^{-1} and 0.84 kg ha^{-1}, respectively, on 24 May. The area within the cage was marked with rows spaced 68.5 cm apart to be used as a guide for planting with push planters.

The seed for the study were planted on 25 May. A susceptible cultivar, 'Centennial' (27), was planted at 27 seed per meter of row in border rows as well as a 1 m section at the ends of each row of experimental material. Seed to produce experimental plants were scarified, treated with metalaxyl, and space planted 25 cm apart. The parents, D86-3429 and Braxton, were planted in three 12.7 m rows for a total of 150 plants each. Also, 50 seed from each of the fourteen BC$_1$ and six BC$_2$ plants were planted in 12.7 m rows. Following the backcross progeny, five F$_1$ seed each of the cross D86-3429 $\times$ Braxton and its reciprocal were planted. These were followed by the 360 F$_2$ seed from the F$_1$ (D86-3429 $\times$ Braxton) plants grown in 1989. The insect-resistant germplasm lines D75-10169 (29) and PI 229358 (83) were planted in the middle and at the end of the experimental material for a total of 70 plants each.

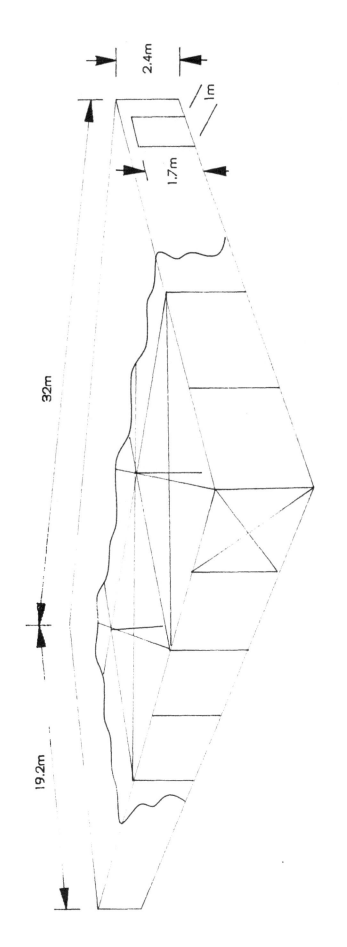

Figure 4. Schematic drawing of field cages used in the 1990 and 1991 experiment.

Normal production practices were used to maintain healthy plants. Soil was cultivated on 7 and 20 June to control weeds, and bentazon [3-(1-methylethyl)-(1H)-2,1,3-benzothiadiazin-4(3H)-one 2,2-dioxide] was applied at 0.84 kg ha^{-1} on 19 June with a hand held pneumatic sprayer. Supplemental irrigation was not required during this time. A Saran cage top (43) was installed on 21 June as the final step in preparation for the release of insects.

Approximately 4000 laboratory-reared (26) soybean looper moths were released in the cage at 0830 h on 25 June. The absence of physical restrictions made all areas of the cage equally accessible to the moths. Water was applied by furrow irrigation to elevate the relative humidity within the cage to enhance egg laying. All plants were at the V5 to V6 growth stage at the time of release. Larvae emerged from eggs after an incubation period of approximately three days.

Larvae were allowed to feed until susceptible Centennial was determined to be 85 to 90 % defoliated which occurred on 6 July or 11 days after moths were released. At that time, methomyl was applied at 0.5 kg ha^{-1} with a backpack sprayer to kill the loopers and stop further feeding. On 9 July, the Saran cage top was removed to facilitate regrowth by plants that were to be harvested for use in 1991, and all plants in the study were evaluated for defoliation. Each plant was assigned a score of 1-to-10 (AV method) based on the visual estimate of defoliation. The 1-to-10 rating scale represented 10% increments, with a score of 1 representing defoliation of 0 to 10% and a score of 10 representing defoliation of 91 to 100%.

Ratings for the two parents, D86-3429 and Braxton, and their F_1 and F_2 progeny were grouped by their defoliation scores and plotted on a graph. The distribution of the parental and F_2 populations were tested for normality following the procedure described by Leonard et al. (49). Initially the defoliation data of these populations were summarized in frequency distributions by using the upper class limits. The mean $\bar{x}$, variance s^2, and standard deviation s of each population were calculated from the class centers (i.e. 0.5, 1.5, 2.5, ... 9.5) using the following formulas:

$$\bar{x} = n_1(0.5) + n_2(1.5) + ... + n_{10}(9.5)/(n_1 + n_2 + ... + n_{10})$$

$$s^2 = n_1(0.5 - \bar{x}) + n_1(1.5 - \bar{x}) + ... + n_1(9.5 - \bar{x})/(n_{..} - 1)$$

$$s = (s^2)^{1/2}$$

where n_n was the number of plants in each of the respective classes and $n_{..}$ was the grand total. Following the calculation of these variables, the variable x was calculated for each class in the following manner:

$$x = (\bar{x} - \text{upper class limit})/s$$

After determining the x for each class, a table of normal probability integrals was used to determine the corresponding Z value of each class. The theoretical percentage of each population was calculated by subtracting Z from 1.000 and multiplying by 100. The theoretical number of each class was calculated as follows:

$$n_{..} \times \text{theoretical } \% = \text{theoretical } n$$

For each succeeding class, the cumulative percentage in all prior classes must be subtracted to obtain the theoretical percentage to calculate the theoretical n of that class. The observed distribution versus theoretical distribution was tested with a X^2 test. This was done to gain insight into the mode of inheritance of resistance to soybean looper and to facilitate the design of the 1991 experiments. The information from these four populations was used to determine what additional crosses, if any, would be required to fulfill the objectives of this study.

The original cross, D86-3429 × Braxton, was repeated to generate seed to be used as the F_1 generation in 1991. The two backcrosses, BC_1 and BC_2, were repeated for the same purpose as the original cross, as well as to provide seed for planting in a winter nursery to generate the BS_1 and BS_2 populations, the selfed generations of the backcrosses. The bulk of the pollinations were made on plants within the cage. The remainder were on plants located in the F_2 nursery. Plants within the cage were irrigated as needed throughout the remainder of the growing season to insure adequate seed set on F_1 and F_2 plants for use the following year.

Twelve seeds were produced from the D86-3429 × Braxton cross. The two backcrosses, BC_1 and BC_2, yielded 49 and 29 seeds, respectively. The 12 F_1 seeds were combined with remnant D86-3429 × Braxton F_1 seed generated from the 1988 and 1989 crosses for use in 1991. Twelve seeds and 11 seeds, from BC_1 and BC_2, respectively, were scarified and treated with metalaxyl and sent to the winter nursery at Mayaguez, Puerto Rico to produce the BS_1 and BS_2 generations. The single plants from the various generations in the cage were harvested and threshed with a single-plant thresher between

31 October and 2 November. The soil in the cage was subsoiled on 9 November in preparation for the 1991 experiment.

<u>1991</u>

Two field cages were used to complete the inheritance study. Soil in each cage was disked with a disk harrow and treated with trifluralin at 0.84 kg ha^{-1}, which was incorporated with a spring-tooth harrow on 26 April. To control a broad spectrum of weeds, a tank mix of clomazone at 1.12 kg ha^{-1} and imazaquin [2-(4,5-dihydro-4-methyl-4-(1-methylethyl)-5-oxo-1H-imidazol-2-yl)-3-quinolinecarboxylic acid] at 0.11 kg ha^{-1} was applied and incorporated with a spring-tooth harrow on 13 May. On 25 May, soil was reworked with a spring-tooth harrow and rows spaced 68.6 cm apart were marked to serve as guides for the push planter.

Each row consisted of 10 plants spaced 25 cm apart except for the F_1, BC_1, and BC_2 generations, which had only one plant per row. There were three rows, consisting of 10 plants each, of the insect-resistant germplasm lines D75-10169 and PI 229358. The planting order for each cage was generated by randomizing the 277 rows with PC-SAS PROC PLAN (68). Each cage contained the entire complement of plants and was treated as a replication over environments.

The border rows were planted to Centennial at 27 seed per meter in each cage. The rows of experimental populations were centered 68.6 cm apart. Rainfall of 43 mm halted planting on 25 May in cage 1 after one third of the rows were planted. The remainder of cage 1 and all of cage 2 was lightly tilled with a spring-tooth harrow on 29 May. The remaining rows in cage 1 were planted on 29 May. Approximately 1 m of

Centennial was planted at the ends of all rows to serve as a border. The experimental populations were surrounded by a susceptible cultivar.

On 31 May, soil in cage 2 was rolled with a water-filled roller pulled by a four-wheel all-terrain vehicle. This operation smoothed and firmed the seed bed, which decreased the rate of evaporation of moisture from the soil. The rows were then marked as in cage 1. The susceptible cultivar Centennial was planted by the same method as in cage 1. The entire area within cage 2 was planted on 31 May. Short sections of the Centennial border rows were replanted on 14 June.

Soil in the cages was cultivated on 4, 14, 20, and 26 June with a self-propelled garden tiller. Supplemental soil moisture was provided by furrow irrigation on 4 and 21 June to ensure that the plants would have sufficient vegetative growth at the time of insect release. The Saran tops were put on the cages on 26 June as final preparation for the release of insects.

Approximately 4000 laboratory-reared (26) soybean looper moths were released in each cage at 0800 h on 8 July. A rainfall of 19 mm on 4 July provided sufficient soil moisture to maintain an elevated relative humidity within the cages during the egg-laying period. At the time of release, the plants were at the V7 to V8 stage of growth in cage 1, and V6 to V7 in cage 2 (17). Larvae emerged after an incubation period of approximately three days.

Larvae were allowed to feed in each cage until 22 July, at which time Centennial was approximately 95% defoliated. The cage tops were then removed to facilitate the defoliation ratings and to promote regrowth of the plants. Both cages were sprayed with methomyl at 0.5 kg ha^{-1} to kill larvae. This insured that additional feeding would not occur once the ratings had begun. Cage 1 was rated on 23 and 24 July using the AV rating method. This method used the same 1-to-10 scale previously described for the WP method in 1990. In the AV method the plants were visually partitioned into three sections (top, middle, bottom). Each section was scored for defoliation and these three scores were averaged to get the mean score for each plant. This method enabled the evaluator to make a more detailed assessment of defoliation by the soybean looper on each plant. Cage 2 was rated during a rainfall by the same method on 25 and 26 July. All ratings in both cages were made by the same evaluator.

Generation means and variances were calculated for each of the nine generations on a cage basis. These means and variances were employed in Mather's scaling tests (51) to determine the adequacy of an additive - dominant model and to test for epistasis. The formulas for the different scaling tests were as follows:

$$A = 2\bar{x}BC_1 - \bar{x}P_1 - \bar{x}F_1 \qquad V_A = 4V\bar{x}BC_1 + V\bar{x}P_1 + V\bar{x}F_1$$

$$B = 2\bar{x}BC_2 - \bar{x}P_2 - \bar{x}F_1 \qquad V_B = 4V\bar{x}BC_2 + V\bar{x}P_2 + V\bar{x}F_1$$

$$C = 4\bar{x}F_2 - 2\bar{x}F_1 - \bar{x}P_1 - \bar{x}P_2 \qquad V_C = 16V\bar{x}F_2 + 4V\bar{x}F_1 + V\bar{x}P_1 + V\bar{x}P_2$$

$$D = 8\bar{x}F_3 - 3\bar{x}P_1 - 3\bar{x}P_2 - 2\bar{x}F_1 \qquad V_D = 64V\bar{x}F_3 + 9V\bar{x}P_1 + 9V\bar{x}P_2 + 4V\bar{x}F_1$$

where $\bar{x}$ was the mean of the respective generations and $V\bar{x}$ was the variance of the mean of the same respective generations. The variance of the mean of each generation was calculated as $V\bar{x} = \sigma^2/n$, where σ^2 was the variance of the generation and n was the number of individuals observed in that generation.

To determine if each of the scaling tests had the expected value of zero, each was tested in the following manner:

$$t_A = A/(V_A)^{\frac{1}{2}}$$

$$t_B = B/(V_B)^{\frac{1}{2}}$$

$$t_C = C/(V_C)^{\frac{1}{2}}$$

$$t_D = D/(V_D)^{\frac{1}{2}}$$

where $(V_A)^{\frac{1}{2}}$, $(V_B)^{\frac{1}{2}}$, $(V_C)^{\frac{1}{2}}$, and $(V_D)^{\frac{1}{2}}$ were the standard errors of each tests. The t values obtained were compared to a table of t distribution (76) to determine the level of significance for each of the tests. The probability was found in the table of t using the sum of the degrees of freedom of each generation in each test as the number of degrees of freedom.

Since the preliminary results indicated that resistance to soybean looper is inherited quantitatively, it was necessary to select an appropriate method of analysis that would allow for a detailed study of the inheritance of resistance. After reviewing the statistical methods available for the analysis of a quantitative trait, a generation means analysis was selected. This analysis was chosen over other methods because of the following advantages (23):

1.   Errors are inherently smaller since means (first order statistics) are used, rather than variances (second order statistics);

2.   Smaller experiments allow the same degree of precision;

3.   Additive (*a*), dominant (*d*), and epistatic (*aa, ad,* and *dd*)

effects are estimated   using means rather than variances;

and

4.   It is applicable to both cross- and self-pollinating crops.

In utilizing the generation means analysis, it is assumed that the parents are homozygous and there is no linkage among genes influencing the trait being studied.   If this assumption is correct and it appears that the trait in question is not quantitatively inherited, these generations can be used to analyze for Mendelian ratios.

Hallauer and Miranda (23) cited the following disadvantages to the generation means analysis:

1.   An estimate of heritability cannot be obtained; and

2.   Genetic advances cannot be predicted because genetic

variances are not available.

Although these disadvantages are inherent to the generation means analysis, they are of little consequence since additional calculations can be made to obtain the variances necessary to estimate heritability.

Generation means analysis, as described by Hayman (31), has been used extensively in other crops such as corn (21,34,70), cotton (*Gossypium hirsutum* L.) (55,56), and wheat (8). In most cases, Gamble's (21) notation is used in conjunction with Hayman's (31) methodology. Generation means analysis apparently has not been used previously in soybean to analyze quantitative traits. Because of the advantages of this analysis, it was chosen to determine the mode of inheritance of resistance to soybean looper.

Populations used were derived from the cross D86-3429 × Braxton (Figure 5). A minimum of six populations are required in a generation means analysis with a six parameter model, but this experiment was expanded to include nine populations. The number of individuals comprising each generation are listed in Table 2. To determine the inheritance of resistance to soybean looper in soybean according to Hayman's (31) model, programs were written in SAS to analyze the data by cage (see Appendix C) and combined over cages where cages were treated as blocks (see Appendix D). Using Hayman's methodology and Gamble's (21) notation, the models for the generation means analysis were as follows:

$$
\begin{aligned}
P_1 &= m + a - d/2 + aa - ad + dd/4 \\
P_2 &= m - a - d/2 + aa + ad + dd/4 \\
F_1 &= m \quad\quad + d/2 \quad\quad\quad\quad + dd/4 \\
F_2 &= m \\
BC_1 &= m + a/2 \quad\quad + aa/4 \\
BC_2 &= m - a/2 \quad\quad + aa/4 \\
F_3 &= m \quad\quad - d/4 \quad\quad\quad\quad + dd/16 \\
BS_1 &= m + a/2 - d/4 + aa/4 - ad/4 + dd/16 \\
BS_2 &= m - a/2 - d/4 + aa/4 + ad/4 + dd/16
\end{aligned}
$$

where m = the overall mean, and a, d, aa, ad, and dd represent the additive, dominance, additive × additive, additive × dominance, and dominance × dominance genetic effects, respectively.

Each SAS program fitted two regression models which were set up using matrix notation according to the procedures outlined by Jennings et al. (34). The first

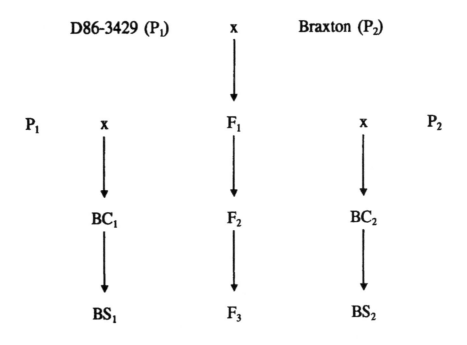

Figure 5. Mating scheme to derive populations required to estimate the genetic effects of resistance to the soybean looper in soybean.

Table 2. Populations used for generation means analysis of the inheritance of resistance to the soybean looper.

Population	Gen.	Row Number	Plants per Row†	Total Plants
D86-3429	P_1	1 - 11	10	110
Braxton	P_2	12 - 22	10	110
D86-3429 × Braxton	F_1	23 - 35	1	13
D86-3429 × Braxton	F_2	36 - 85	1	500
D86-3429 × Braxton	F_3	86 - 210	10	1250
D86-3429(2) × Braxton	BC_1	211 - 224	1	14
D86-3429(2) × Braxton	BS_1	225 - 249	10	250
Braxton(2) × D86-3429	BC_2	250 - 255	1	6
Braxton(2) × D86-3429	BS_2	256 - 271	10	160
D75-10169‡	-	272 - 274	10	30
PI 229358‡	-	275 - 277	10	30

†Rows were 2.5 cm long except where there was only 1 plant/row.
‡Insect-resistant germplasm lines used as checks.

regression model, defined as Model 1, consisted of the three parameters m, a, and d. The second regression model, defined as Model 2, consisted of the epistatic effects, aa, ad, and dd, in addition to the parameters in Model 1. Model 2 is used only if a significant additive or dominant effect is detected and to determine if significant epistatic effects exist that are contributing to the significance in Model 1. To adjust for the unequal population sizes comprising each generation, the models were weighted using reciprocals of the standard errors of the generation means as suggested by Rowe and Alexander (65).

In addition, Powers' partitioning method of genetic analysis (49,61) was incorporated to test proposed genetic models. Initially the frequency distributions of the P_1, P_2, F_1, and F_2 generations were tested for normality by testing the observed versus theoretical distribution with a X^2 test following the procedure previously outlined. Frequency distributions (observed and theoretical) of the F_2 population were converted to percentages in each class in the following manner:

$$\%(\text{in each class}) = n_i/n_{..}$$

where n_i was the number of plants in each class and $n_{..}$ was the total number of plants in the F_2 population. After conversion, the observed distribution of the F_2 population was examined for modes. Finally, the F_2 population of each cage was tested for goodness of fit to a two-gene additive model. The proposed genetic ratio for the model was as follows: 1:2:1:2:4:2:1:2:1. To test the model, the ratio was simplified to 1:14:1 by combining the defoliation classes in the two cages as follows: 2-4, 5-8, and 9-10 in cage 1, and 2-3, 4-8, and 9-10 in cage 2. The end classes were defined by a distinct transition between defoliation class in the distribution of the F_2 population of each cage.

The homozygous populations D86-3429, Braxton, D75-10169, and PI 229358 were used to determine if there was a significant location effect within each cage. An analysis of variance was performed on each population to obtain the row and plant within row mean squares. Estimates for plant to plant variability within a row (σ^2_p) and the additional variability of plants in different rows (σ^2_r) were obtained from the expected values of the mean squares. Also, F-tests for significant row effects $(H_0:\sigma^2_r=0)$ were performed on each of the homozygous generations within each cage.

An estimate for the number of genes (n) involved in resistance to soybean looper was obtained for the progeny in each cage by the formula:

$$n = (\bar{x}P_1 - \bar{x}P_2)^2/8[(\sigma^2F_2) - ((v_1\sigma^2P_1+v_2\sigma^2P_2+v_3\sigma^2F_1)/v_1+v_2+v_3)]$$

In the formula, $\bar{x}P_1$ and $\bar{x}P_2$, were the mean defoliation ratings for the parents, and σ^2F_2, σ^2P_1, σ^2P_2, and σ^2F_1 were the variances of the respective generations. This formula is a modification of the formula presented by Poehlman (60). In the modification, σ^2F_1 is replaced with $(v_1\sigma^2P_1+v_2\sigma^2P_2+v_3\sigma^2F_1)/(v_1+v_2+v_3)$. This modification was used in order to better estimate the environmental variance, since σ^2F_1, σ^2P_1, and σ^2P_2 were essentially estimates of environmental variation. The degrees of freedom (v_1, v_2, and v_3) for the associated generations were employed to lessen population size effects on the estimate of environmental variance. This method of estimating genes assumes that the genes have equal effects without significant dominant or epistatic effects.

Heritability of insect resistance, in the broad sense, was estimated for the progeny

in each cage from the formula:

$$H = (V_G/V_P) \times 100\%$$

where V_G was the genetic variance and V_P was the phenotypic variance. The genetic

variance was:

$$V_G = V_P - V_E$$

where V_E was the environmental variance. The V_E was estimated by obtaining the

weighted average of the variances of the F_1 population and the populations of the parents

P_1 and P_2:

$$(v_1\sigma^2P_1 + v_2\sigma^2P_2 + v_3\sigma^2F_1)/(v_1 + v_2 + v_3)$$

In the formula the respective degrees of freedom v were used to weight the variances of

each population. The V_P was estimated by utilizing the variance of the F_2 population.

Results and Discussion

1990

The defoliation data of the P_1, P_2, F_1, and F_2 populations from the preliminary

cage study are presented in Table 3. Also presented in this table are the defoliation

ratings of PI 229358 and D75-10169, from which D86-3429 derived its resistance to

soybean looper. D86-3429 was visibly more resistant than the original source of

Table 3. Ratings of leaf feeding by soybean looper on soybean parents, their F_1 and F_2 progeny, and the germplasm lines PI 229358 and D75-10169 in the field cage-1990.

	\multicolumn{11}{c}{Upper class limits of leaf feeding ratings†}										
	1	2	3	4	5	6	7	8	9	$\bar{x}$	n
D86-3429(P_1)	4	60	64	11						2.6	139
Braxton(P_2)				1	32	48	38	19	1	6.3	139
$P_1 \times P_2$(F_1)			5							3.0	5
$P_2 \times P_1$(F_1)			1	4						3.8	5
$P_1 \times P_2$(F_2)	1	33	78	154	39	6	2	1		3.7	314
PI 229358			21	25	1	1				3.6	48
D75-10169		4	34	18						3.3	56

†1 = 0 to 10% defoliation, 2 = 11 to 20%, 3 = 21 to 30%, 4 = 31 to 40%, 5 = 41 to 50%, 6 = 51 to 60%, 7 = 61 to 70%, 8 = 71 to 80%, 9 = 81 to 90%, 10 = 91 to 100%. None of the plants received a rating of 10.

resistance, PI 229358. This suggests that additional genes for resistance might be contributing to the increased level of resistance.

Resistance to soybean looper was interpreted as being quantitatively inherited based on the defoliation data of the P_1, P_2, F_1, and F_2 populations (Table 3). Distribution of the F_2 population (n=314) was continuous, with a mean defoliation rating of 3.7 which was slightly less than the parental midpoint of 4.5. Although a high number of individuals fell in the fourth rating class (31 to 40% defoliation), the F_2 population appeared to have a normal distribution. The P_1, P_2, and F_2 population distributions were tested for normality using the procedure outlined by Leonard et al. (49) (see Appendix E). Both parental populations had low X^2 values (Table 4) indicating they were normally distributed. The frequency distribution of the F_2 ratings failed the normal distribution test (Table 4). Rating class 4 had too many plants, whereas classes 3 and 5 had too few (Table 3 and Appendix E).

Although the defoliation ratings of the F_2 population did not fit a normal curve the distribution was continuous with only one mode. Therefore use of a method of data analysis for quantitative traits seemed appropriate in order to define the mode of inheritance of soybean looper resistance. A generation means analysis (31,34) was chosen and additional crosses were made to supply the generations necessary for the experiment.

1991

Larvae were allowed to feed until susceptible Centennial was 95% defoliated. Plants were found in all rating classes except class one. All populations receiving larger

Table 4. Goodness of fit test for normality† of soybean looper defoliation for populations of D86-3429, Braxton, and D86-3429 x Braxton F_2 populations in the 1990 cage study.

Population	Degrees of Freedom	X^2	P
D86-3429	3	3.6628	0.50 - 0.25
Braxton	5	7.1877	0.50 - 0.25
F_2	7	22.3204	< 0.005

† Test follows the procedure of Leonard et al. (49).

mean defoliation scores in 1991 (Table 5) than in 1990 (Table 3), when larvae were killed when Centennial was only 85% defoliated.

In 1991 the AV rating method was substituted for the WP method used in 1990. The AV method accounted for feeding preferences of soybean looper (24). It was expected to yield a better estimate of defoliation than the WP method, because each score of the AV method was the average of three observations per plant, whereas the WP method was based on a single observation. The AL method was too time consuming to be used in an experiment of this magnitude with the resources available.

Ratings of defoliation by soybean looper on the parents, P_1 and P_2, and their F_1, F_2, and F_3 progenies grown in cages 1 and 2 are shown in Table 5. The F_2 and F_3 progenies, in both cages, exhibited a normal distribution for ratings of defoliation. In both cages the F_1 population exhibited a bimodal distribution instead of the expected single mode. All of the F_1 plants exhibited purple flowers and tawny pubescence, ruling out the possibility that the bimodal distribution resulted from selfs in D86-3429.

The F_1 defoliation data distribution was expected to exhibit a narrow range and single mode intermediate to the two parental modes. Instead the distribution had a wide range and was bimodal in both cages (Table 5). Since the F_1 data did not fit expected distributions, it was suspected that there was a location effect within each cage interfering with the defoliation ratings. The four homozygous populations (D86-3429, Braxton, D75-10169, and PI 229358) included in the study were tested to determine if there was a significant location effect within each cage. A significant location effect was detected for the populations of D86-3429, Braxton, and D75-10169 in each cage (Table 6).

Table 5. Ratings of leaf feeding by soybean looper on soybean parents, their F_1, F_2, F_3, BC_1, BS_1, BC_2, and BS_2 progeny, and the germplasm lines PI 229358 and D75-10169 in the field cages-1991.

| | Upper Class Limits of Leaf feeding ratings† | | | | | | | | | | |
	2	3	4	5	6	7	8	9	10	x̄‡	n
					Cage 1						
D86-3429(P_1)	3	30	44	19	2					3.5	98
Braxton(P_2)					2	18	30	40	4	8.0	94
$P_1 \times P_2(F_1)$		1	2		2	6				5.8	11
$P_1 \times P_2(F_2)$	1	8	31	58	102	111	67	36	4	6.2	418
$P_1 \times P_2(F_3)$	7	37	118	194	232	201	148	131	18	6.0	1086
P_1 x (P_1 x P_2)(BC_1)		5	4	1	1	1	2			4.4	14
P_1 x (P_1 x P_2)(BS_1)	2	34	64	61	19	8	6			4.2	194
P_2 x (P_1 x P_2)(BC_2)							3	1		7.9	4
P_2 x (P_1 x P_2)(BS_2)			1		10	13	52	45	9	7.9	130
PI 229358		1	1	7	11	1				5.1	21
D75-10169	2	7	10	7	2					3.6	28
					Cage 2						
D86-3429(P_1)	8	32	43	14						3.3	97
Braxton(P_2)			1			5	34	43	11	8.3	94
$P_1 \times P_2(F_1)$	1	2	1		2	3	2	1		5.4	12
$P_1 \times P_2(F_2)$	2	17	43	58	82	120	93	30	5	6.1	450
$P_1 \times P_2(F_3)$		28	103	189	238	273	187	114	21	6.2	1153
P_1 x (P_1 x P_2)(BC_1)		2	5	3	2	2				4.5	14
P_1 x (P_1 x P_2)(BS_1)	5	23	59	51	37	16	7	1		4.5	199
P_2 x (P_1 x P_2)(BC_2)									2	9.3	2
P_2 x (P_1 x P_2)(BS_2)			1	5	12	17	33	43	11	7.7	122
PI 229358			3	16	8	1				4.9	28
D75-10169		3	9	9	6					4.4	27

†Based on the mean of three observations per plant. 1 = 0 to 10% defoliation, 2 = 11 to 20%, 3 = 21 to 30%, 4 = 31 to 40%, 5 = 41 to 50%, 6 = 51 to 60%, 7 = 61 to 70%, 8 = 71 to 80%, 9 = 81 to 90%, 10 = 91 to 100%. None of the plants received a rating of 1.
‡Derived from the mean defoliation of all plants without regard of the upper class limits.

Table 6. Estimates of variance components obtained from an analysis of the homogeneous populations, D86-3429, Braxton, D75-10169, PI 229358, for a location effect due to feeding[†] by soybean looper in field cages in 1991.

Population	σ^2_p[‡]	$\sigma^2_p + \sigma^2_r$[§]	F $H_0 : \sigma^2_r = 0$
Cage 1			
D86-3429 (P$_1$)	0.31	0.72	12.55***
Braxton (P$_2$)	0.25	0.84	20.78***
D75-10169 (BD)	0.29	1.50	40.29***
PI 229358 (D)	0.58	0.96	5.37*
Cage 2			
D86-3429 (P$_1$)	0.37	0.54	5.03***
Braxton (P$_2$)	0.69	0.80	2.35*
D75-10169 (BD)	0.42	0.94	12.03***
PI 229358 (D)	0.39	0.41	1.41

*, *** Significant at the 0.05 and 0.001 probability levels respectively.

[†] Based on defoliation ratings made with a 1 to 10 scale divided into 10% increments with a 10 reflecting 91-100% damage.

[‡] Variance of plants within same row.

[§] Variance of plants among rows.

The location effect for the PI 229358 population was significant (p < 0.05, Table 6) in cage 1, but was nonsignificant in cage 2. Although the population size of PI 229358 is approximately the same for each cage, different randomization plans would produce different results. It is apparent that the defoliation ratings were affected by location within the cages.

The mean ratings for soybean looper defoliation and their standard errors for the nine generations grown in each cage are presented in Table 7. In addition to the observed mean ratings for defoliation, the predicted means determined from relationships described by Mather and Jinks (51) are also presented. In all instances except the BC_2 generation in cage 2, the predicted means were within $\pm$ one standard deviation of the observed means in each cage. The observed mean for the BC_2 generation in each cage was larger than the predicted mean. This deviation from the predicted mean could be associated with the small sample size available for defoliation ratings. Variances of the generations from each cage are presented in Table 7, and are used later in Mather's scaling test (51) and to determine heritability.

The results of Mather's scaling test (51) for the cross D86-3429 x Braxton are shown in Table 8. According to Mather and Jinks (51), if the values of A, B, C, and D do not differ from zero, then additive gene effects are indicated. The significance of any of these scales indicates the presence of epistasis. In cage 1, nonsignificant values for A, B, C, and D, indicated that an additive-dominance model was adequate. Cage 2 data yielded similar t-tests for A, C, and D, supporting the conclusions from cage 1. The B scale test could not be applied to cage 2 since the BC_2 population had a variance

Table 7. Means, standard errors, and variances of soybean looper defoliation ratings for parental lines and seven populations of soybean arising from the cross D86-3429 × Braxton grown in field cages at Stoneville, MS in 1991.

| Population | Gen. | Number | Mean | | S.E.‡ | σ^2 |
			Actual	Pred†		
Cage 1						
D86-3429	P_1	98	3.49	-	0.084	0.685
Braxton	P_2	94	7.97	-	0.092	0.797
$P_1 \times P_2$	F_1	11	5.76	5.73	0.427	2.002
$P_1 \times P_2$	F_2	418	6.19	5.75	0.072	2.160
$P_1 \times P_2$	F_3	1086	6.02	5.96	0.052	2.916
$P_1 \times (P_1 \times P_2)$	BC_1	14	4.36	4.63	0.524	3.837
$P_1 \times (P_1 \times P_2)$	BS_1	194	4.22	4.62	0.087	1.452
$P_2 \times (P_1 \times P_2)$	BC_2	4	7.92	6.87	0.394	0.620
$P_2 \times (P_1 \times P_2)$	BS2	130	7.89	6.86	0.090	1.055
Cage 2						
D86-3429	P_1	97	3.34	-	0.074	0.528
Braxton	P_2	94	8.28	-	0.092	0.788
$P_1 \times P_2$	F_1	12	5.42	5.81	0.617	4.568
$P_1 \times P_2$	F_2	450	6.13	5.62	0.074	2.490
$P_1 \times P_2$	F_3	1153	6.18	5.97	0.046	2.478
$P_1 \times (P_1 \times P_2)$	BC_1	14	4.45	4.38	0.376	1.976
$P_1 \times (P_1 \times P_2)$	BS_1	199	4.52	4.48	0.093	1.708
$P_2 \times (P_1 \times P_2)$	BC_2	2	9.33	6.85	0.000	0.000
$P_2 \times (P_1 \times P_2)$	BS_2	122	7.69	6.95	0.117	1.655

†Based on relationships described by Mather and Jinks, 1971.
‡Standard error

Table 8. Mather's scaling test applied to the cross D86-3429 x Braxton to test adequacy of additive-dominance model for resistance to soybean looper.

Test	Cage 1	Cage 2
t_A	-0.125	0.039
t_B	0.918	-
t_C	0.268	0.267
t_D	0.157	0.273

of zero. Since C was not significantly different from zero in either cage (Table 8), this indicated that generation means depended only on the additive gene effects and no epistasis was present.

The results of the generation means analysis of each cage are reported in Table 9. Table 10 reports the results of the combined analysis where the cage effects are treated as blocks. Significant negative additive effects were detected with Model 1, which measures only additive and dominant effects, for both Cages 1 and 2 ($p < 0.06$ and $p < 0.02$, respectively; Table 9) and the combined cages ($p < 0.001$, Table 10). The sign of this effect is dependent upon the parent designated as P_1. The sign of the effect is a function of the fact that an inverted scale was used and also a reflection of the relationship between the mid-parent and the means of the F_1, F_2, and F_3 generations indicating which parent was contributing to the additive variation (51). In Cage 1 (Table 7) the means of the F_1, F_2, and F_3 generations were between the mid-parent (5.73) and P_2. The means of the F_2 and F_3 in Cage 2 were skewed away from the mid-parent (5.81) in the same direction, but the F_1 mean was oriented towards the other parent. Although the F_1's mean was on the opposite side, it was within one standard deviation of the mean. All of the progeny means skewed towards P_2, in addition to a significant negative additive effect indicated that Braxton might be contributing to the additive variation. Since it has been reported that Braxton does have some level of resistance (64), it stands to reason that it would contribute to the additive effect.

The full model, Model 2, was then fitted to estimate the epistatic effects as well as the remaining additive and dominant effects. None of the epistatic (*aa*, *ad*, and *dd*),

Table 9. Estimates of the additive, dominant, and epistatic effects in the generation means for defoliation by soybean looper in the nine populations of the D86-3429 × Braxton material grown in the field cages at Stoneville, MS in 1991.

Effects	Estimate	Standard error	t value
Cage 1			
Model 1			
F$_2$ mean (m)	5.503	0.655	8.399***
Additive (a)	-1.830	0.805	-2.273†
Dominance (d)	-1.287	2.071	-0.621
Model 2			
F$_2$ mean (m)	5.839	0.775	7.538**
Additive (a)	0.859	2.525	0.340
Dominance (d)	-2.639	3.103	-0.851
Additive × Additive (aa)	-2.182	2.642	-0.826
Additive × Dominance (ad)	3.212	2.737	1.174
Dominance × Dominance (dd)	3.484	9.370	0.372
Cage 2			
Model 1			
F$_2$ mean (m)	5.387	0.575	9.374***
Additive (a)	-2.206	0.667	-3.308*
Dominance (d)	-1.385	1.796	-0.771
Model 2			
F$_2$ mean (m)	5.613	0.590	9.507**
Additive (a)	-0.031	1.929	-0.016
Dominance (d)	-2.673	2.525	-1.059
Additive × Additive (aa)	-2.191	1.953	-1.122
Additive × Dominance (ad)	2.534	2.063	1.228
Dominance × Dominance (dd)	4.302	7.742	0.556

*, **, *** Significant at the 0.05, 0.01, and 0.001 probability levels,respectively.
† Significant at the 0.06 probability level.

Table 10. Estimates of the additive, dominant, and epistatic effects in the generation means for defoliation by soybean looper in the nine populations of the D86-3429 × Braxton material grown in the field cages at Stoneville, MS in 1991.

Effects	Estimate	Standard error	t value
Cages 1 and 2 Combined			
Model 1			
F_2 mean (m)	5.414	0.503	10.760***
Additive (a)	-2.020	0.487	-4.150***
Dominance (d)	-1.327	1.281	-1.040
Model 2			
F_2 mean (m)	5.690	0.418	13.630***
Additive (a)	0.424	1.165	0.360
Dominance (d)	-2.669	1.468	-1.820
Additive × Additive (aa)	-2.195	1.197	-1.830
Additive × Dominance (ad)	2.883	1.254	2.300*
Dominance × Dominance (dd)	3.900	4.464	0.870

*,*** Significant at the 0.05 and 0.001 probability levels, respectively.

additive, or dominant effects were significantly different from zero in either cage. Although unexpected, *ad* was significant (p < 0.05) in the combined analysis and neither the additive or dominant effects were significant. It is interesting and informative that *ad* effect is significant. However, it introduces a dimension that cannot be examined further with currently available data. In Model 1 the epistatic effects are included in the additive effects. For this reason, Model 1 will be assumed to treat the data adequately.

With an indication that inheritance of resistance to soybean looper was controlled by an additive genetic system, the data from each cage were tested to fit a two-gene model. Since no modes were evident in the F_2 or F_3 populations in either cage (Table 5), Power's partitioning analysis was employed to analyze the data and test the predicted gene models following the examples of Deren and Quesenberry (12) and Sage and de Isturiz (67).

Initially, the frequency distributions of the defoliation data from the parental, F_1, and F_2 populations from each cage were tested for normality (Table 11). As was seen in 1990, both parental populations had low X^2 values which indicated that these populations were normally distributed about a central mean. In cage 1, the F_1 population did not have a normal distribution, but the F_2 population's distribution did fit the normal curve. The opposite situation occurred with the F_1 and F_2 populations in cage 2. The differences between the two cages with respect to the F_1 and F_2 populations may be due to a location effect present within the cages.

In the hypothesized two-gene additive model the middle classes were combined resulting in three classes for the model to be tested. Partitioning the middle classes

Table 11. Goodness of fit test for normality of soybean looper defoliation data from 1991 cage study.

Population	Degrees of Freedom	X^2	P
		Cage 1	
D86-3429	4	1.519	0.90 - 0.75
Braxton	4	7.767	0.25 - 0.10
F_1	3	10.667	0.025 - 0.010
F_2	8	6.528	0.75 - 0.50
		Cage 2	
D86-3429	3	0.211	0.990 - 0.975
Braxton	4	4.584	0.500 - 0.250
F_1	6	4.000	0.75 - 0.50
F_2	8	26.599	0.005 >

would have been arbitrary, whereas the end class ratios were easily manipulated to test the model. The F_2 data for each cage were tested for goodness of fit to the ratio of 1:14:1 for the two-gene model. The chi-square probabilities were as follows: cage 1, $0.005 > p$; and cage 2, $0.10 > p > 0.05$. These probabilities are reflective of the test for normality of the F_2 defoliation data in both cages as shown in Table 11. The higher the probability of a normal distribution of the F_2 defoliation data, the lower the probability that the F_2 defoliation data fit the two-gene model. Neither F_2 population fit the two-gene model well. The three-gene model gave a better fit. However, because there is good reason to believe that the scores assigned in this experiment should not be assumed to correspond to genotype effects, the Power's partitioning analysis probably has no utility in these analyses.

An estimate for the number of genes, n, in this cross contributing to the expression of resistance to soybean looper was obtained for both cages using a modification of the formula presented by Poehlman (60). The number of genes contributing to the expression of resistance to the soybean looper in the cross D86-3429 x Braxton was estimated at $n = 1.87$ and $n = 1.91$, cages 1 and 2, respectively.

Broad sense heritability was estimated for resistance to soybean looper in the progeny from both cages. Although it has already been concluded that resistance to soybean looper is controlled by additive gene action, narrow-sense heritabilities could not be calculated because of the size and variances of the BC_1 and BC_2 populations in each cage. Although broad sense heritabilities were calculated, it is assumed that these heritabilities are attributed to only the additive genetic variance and are in fact narrow-sense heritabilities. Since the F_1 generations in both cages exhibited a bimodal distribution for defoliation scores, the environmental variance was estimated by the following formula:

$$(v_{P_1}\sigma^2P_1 + v_{P_2}\sigma^2P_2 + v_{F_1}\sigma^2F_1)/(v_{P_1} + v_{P_2} + v_{F_1})$$

as was done in estimating the number of genes. This gives a better estimate of the environmental variance than just using the σ^2F_1 because the number of individuals comprising the parental generations were relatively large (Table 5). Also, parents are genetically uniform and should only exhibit variability due to the environment. The heritabilities were estimated at 62.3% for cage 1 and 64.3% for cage 2. As has been demonstrated in all previous analyses the results from the two cage studies are in agreement for the estimate of broad sense heritability. Based on the high heritabilities for resistance to soybean looper, it is apparent that the phenotypes expressed in this population were determined by the genetic variation more than by the environmental variation.

Although the estimates for both cages are in agreement, the estimate is probably an underestimation of the total number of genes contributing to soybean looper resistance because these data only estimate the number of genes controlling soybean looper resistance by which D86-3429 and Braxton differ. In both cages, Braxton exhibited a low level of resistance with 80% defoliation, whereas Centennial was almost completely defoliated. When compared to Centennial, which is known for its high susceptibility (47), Braxton has repeatedly demonstrated 15 to 20% less defoliation. Since the inception of this study, resistance of Braxton to foliar-feeding insects has been documented by Rowan et al. (64) in a study to compare the resistance of 46 recommended soybean cultivars in Maturity Groups V, VI, VII, and VIII. In that study, Braxton was cited as being one of the most resistant cultivars in Maturity Group VII.

As in 1990, the insect-resistant germplasm lines, PI 229358 and D75-10169, were included in both cages to provide additional checks and to document the level of resistance in the resistant parent, D86-3429. In both cages, D86-3429 was visibly and statistically (Table 12) more resistant than the original source of resistance, PI 229358. D86-3429 also exhibited more resistance than did D75-10169 in both cages, although it was significantly different at p = 0.01 (LSD) only in cage 2 (Table 12). This suggests that during the five cycles of crossing and selection that occurred in the development of D86-3429 from PI 229358, additional genes were gained from 'Tracy-M', a parent in the fourth cycle. Tracy-M has subsequently been identified as being measurably resistant to foliar-feeding insects (47).

Summary and Conclusions

This research was conducted to determine the mode of inheritance of resistance to soybean looper in soybean. The results from Mather's scaling test (51) applied to the data from each cage study indicated that generation means depend only on the additive gene effects for resistance to soybean looper. Utilizing Hayman's (31) methodology in terms of the generation-means analysis to analyze the data from each cage separately, only the additive genetic effects were significant. When the data from the two cages were combined for analysis the *ad* epistatic effect was significant ($t = 2.30$, $p < 0.005$). However, the primary effect is assumed to be additive based on the results of the analysis

Table 12. Average defoliation scores in soybean populations resistant to soybean looper in 1991 cage study.

Population	n	Mean†
Cage 1		
D86-3429	98	3.49 a
D75-10169	28	3.64 a
PI 229358	21	5.13 b
Cage 2		
D86-3429	97	3.34 a
D75-10169	27	4.35 b
PI 229358	28	5.42 b

† Means followed by the same letter are not significantly different at the $p = 0.01$ (LSD).

of the data from cage 1 ($t = -2.273$, p < 0.06), cage 2 ($t = -3.308$, p < 0.05), and combined ($t = -4.15$, p < 0.001), as was indicated by the scaling test. When Power's partition analysis (49,61) was applied to the data from each cages the F_2 data did not fit a two-gene additive model for resistance to soybean looper.

A modification of Poehlman's (60) formula for determination of gene number was used to estimate the number of genes controlling soybean looper resistance by which the parents D86-3429 and Braxton differ. Two genes were estimated to contribute to the expression of resistance to soybean looper in this cross. Since the formula used only estimates the number of genes in which the two parents, the actual number of genes for resistance to soybean looper is probably greater than two. It would take further research with PI 229358 and/or its derived breeding lines to determine exactly how many genes are controlling resistance to soybean looper. Also, the information generated from this research could be integrated with the results of research involving other sources of resistance (36,45,54,72,83) to determine the number of genes that not only control resistance to soybean looper, but other insect species as well.

Heritability was estimated to be 63% for resistance to soybean looper. Broad sense heritabilities were calculated because the size and variances of the BC_1 and BC_2 populations were insufficient, thus prohibiting calculation of narrow-sense heritability. The previous analyses suggests that resistance to soybean looper in this cross is controlled by two genes which behave additively, therefore it can be assumed that this heritability is due only to the additive genetic variance. Since the genetic variation influences resistance to soybean looper more than environmental variation, a breeder should be able to make selections in the F_2 population with confidence.

By utilizing a population from a cross between a resistant breeding line and a highly susceptible breeding line, it should be possible to determine if there are only three genes for resistance to soybean looper in breeding lines derived from PI 229358. The single seed descent method of breeding (60) could be used to determine the number of genes involved by advancing a large population to the F_6 generation and evaluating replicated hills for reaction to soybean looper. For example, assuming three segregating gene pairs, 91% of the F_6 lines should be homozygous (6) for their respective genotypes, thus allowing for replications of each genotype. Replicating the F_6 lines, as well as their parents, increases the precision and accuracy of the measured reaction to soybean looper for each genotype. Examination of results from this type of experiment should indicate whether or not there are only three genes controlling resistance to soybean looper.

Another way to determine if there are only three genes for resistance to soybean looper in PI 229358 derived genotypes would be to utilize restriction fragment length polymorphism (RFLP) markers. RFLP markers have been widely used in other plant species to construct linkage maps and to place genes that control qualitative and quantitative traits onto these maps. Recently, RFLP markers have been used to map phytophthora resistance loci in soybean (13). This methodology could be used to map the genes and possibly determine any linkage groups that may be associated with the genes controlling resistance to soybean looper.

Since the results of this study have shown that resistance to soybean looper was a quantitative trait that was additive, it should be possible to increase the level of resistance in future breeding lines. This might be accomplished by utilizing new sources of resistance which have additional genes for insect resistance. Another method of increasing the level of resistance to soybean looper would be by interspecific hybridization which would allow genes for resistance in other species to be incorporated into the soybean plant.

To fully exploit the benefits of insect resistant breeding lines, it will become necessary to understand the mechanisms of resistance that the plants possess. Depending on the source of resistance, the mechanism of resistance may be different in the various sources. Several researchers (39,53,63,73,81) have already conducted studies on the mechanisms of resistance, but further research is needed. As new technology becomes available, the mysteries of the mechanisms of insect resistance and the genes that control their expression are closer to being solved.

CHAPTER 5
SUMMARY AND CONCLUSIONS

Soybean is grown worldwide primarily for its oil and meal products, and to a lesser degree the whole bean product. As in any crop, soybean is exposed to biotic and abiotic yield-reducing factors such as diseases, nematodes, insects, and drought throughout the growing season. To produce a profitable crop a grower must modify the effects of these yield-reducing factors by one or more of the methods described by Metcalf and Luckmann (50). Environmentally, the best approach to any pest problem would be to utilize genes for resistance in available germplasm to develop resistant cultivars (82).

Soybean looper is a major pest to soybean in many areas of the southeastern United States. The soybean looper, more so than any other arthropod pest, has become increasingly resistant to available insecticides (10,18,48,58,60) making it difficult to control. By utilizing soybean germplasm lines that possess genes for resistance to foliar-feeding insects, it is possible to increase the host plant responses for control as has been demonstrated by the development of the insect-resistant cultivars Lamar (28) and Crockett (5).

The objectives of this study were: (*i*) to evaluate three methods of rating for defoliation of soybean by soybean looper, and (*ii*) to determine the inheritance of resistance in soybean to the soybean looper. The latter was the most important objective since knowledge of inheritance of a particular trait increases the efficiency for incorporating genes for that trait into an agronomically desirable plant type. Rating methodology can affect the accuracy of classification and therefore was evaluated separately to offer guidelines for future insect defoliation studies.

Evaluation of Rating Methods

The three methods of defoliation assessment evaluated in 1990 and 1991 were the whole plant visual rating (WP), the partitioned plant average visual rating (AV), and measured average leaf area of the partitioned plant (AL). The WP and AV were visual assessments of defoliation based on a 1-to-10 scale divided into 10% increments with a score of 1 signifying defoliation of 0 to 10% and a score of 10 signifying defoliation of 91 to 100%. The WP method was based on one observation per plant, whereas the AV method was based on the mean of three observations per plants. The absolute method (AL) utilized a LI-COR LI-3000 leaf area meter to measure the area of three trifoliolates, one each from the top, middle, and bottom of the plant.

In 1990 no absolute method comparisons were possible, however the WP and AV were highly correlated ($r=0.65$, $p < 0.001$). Adjustments in the method of calculating percent defoliation by AL for 1991 allowed for direct comparisons with the WP and AV methods. All correlations (WP vs. AV, WP vs. AL, and AV vs. AL) were significant at the $p < 0.001$ level whether the cages were examined separately or pooled. The results of these correlations indicate that the evaluator could obtain similar estimates of defoliation regardless of which of the three methods is utilized. These findings are similar to the results of another relative versus absolute estimation of defoliation study conducted in 1985 by G.R. Bowers (G.R. Bowers, 1992, personal communication).

A paired difference comparison was performed to test the equality of the defoliation assessment between the relative methods in 1990 and among the three methods in 1991. The results indicated that estimates of defoliation by the two relative methods in 1990 and by all three in 1991 were significantly different. With the relative methods, WP and AV, the evaluator estimated somewhat similar amounts of defoliation across all plants when compared with each other, even though the difference between the two methods was highly significant. However, in comparisons with an absolute method, as in 1991, it becomes apparent that the evaluator's estimates of defoliation with the WP method were closer to the actual than were the estimates of the AV method. These findings were validated with McNemar's test for concordance.

The relative variation (RV) was calculated for each method as a measure of precision. In 1990 the precision of the WP and AV methods were essentially equal. Similar results were obtained in 1991 by all three methods. Both years the precision of the methods was essentially equal and well below 10, the value that Pedigo states as being desirable in research. These results indicate that either relative method, WP or AV, would be suitable for estimating defoliation by insects.

Based on the results of these studies it is apparent that relative estimates of defoliation can be used in genetic studies or routine screenings of advanced breeding lines, in lieu of an absolute estimate. Since the two relative methods yielded similar results it would advantageous to use the simplest and most economical method for making estimates of defoliation. With increased experience in visual estimates of defoliation, researchers should be able to estimate defoliation with reliability and repeatability.

Inheritance Study

This study was undertaken to determine the mode of inheritance of resistance to the soybean looper in soybean. The study consisted of two years of field cage evaluations of progeny derived from the cross D86-3429 x Braxton. The results of the preliminary study in 1990 suggested that the genes controlling resistance to soybean looper might be inherited quantitatively. The 1991 experiment was designed so that inheritance of resistance to soybean looper could be examined quantitatively as well as qualitatively. Also, the 1991 experiment was duplicated in two field cages so that the experiment would be repeated in two separate environments to strengthen the results and conclusions of the study.

In the 1991 study, estimates of defoliation were made for each plant using the AV method. Although this method was more time consuming than the WP method, it was chosen because its estimate of defoliation was based on three observations per plant rather than one observation. After assessing each plant in each cage for defoliation by the soybean looper the data generated were analyzed by several methods of genetic analysis.

Mather's scaling test (51) was applied to the defoliation data from each cage study and it was determined that generation means depend only on the additive gene effects and no epistasis was present. Utilizing Hayman's (31) methodology in terms of the generation-means analysis to analyze the data from each cage separately, only the additive genetic effects were significant. When the data from the two cages were combined for analysis the *ad* epistatic effect was significant ($t = 2.30$, $p < 0.005$). However, the primary effect is assumed to be additive based on the results of the analysis of the data from cage 1 ($t = -2.273$, $p < 0.06$), cage 2 ($t = -3.308$, $p < 0.05$), and combined ($t = -4.15$, $p < 0.001$), as was indicated by the scaling test. Applying Power's partitioning analysis (49,61) to the data from each cage it was determined that in this cross the F_2 data did not fit the two-gene additive model for resistance to soybean looper. There is good reason to believe that the defoliation scores assigned in this experiment should not be assumed to correspond to genotype effects, therefore the Power's partitioning analysis has no utility in these analyses.

Based on a modification of the formula presented by Poehlman (60), it was determined that two genes contribute to the expression of resistance to soybean looper in this cross. However this formula only estimates the number of genes for resistance to soybean looper by which the two parents differ. In actuality the number of genes for resistance to soybean looper is probably greater than two, but it would take further research to determine this.

Broad sense heritability based on the defoliation data was estimated to be 63% for resistance to soybean looper. Since the previous analyses suggest that resistance to the soybean looper is controlled by two genes which behave additively, it can be assumed that this heritability is due only to the additive genetic variation. A heritability of this magnitude suggests that a breeder should be able to make progress by selecting for resistance to soybean looper in early generations.

This research could be continued with breeding lines derived from PI 229358 or by incorporating additional sources of resistance, such as PI 227687, PI 171451, PI 417061, or PI 507301 into agronomically adapted breeding lines. These elite genotypes could then be cross-pollinated with a highly susceptible cultivar, such as Centennial, to develop large F_2 populations for future evaluations. In order to determine the number of genes controlling resistance to the soybean looper and/or other species, these F_2 populations could be screened by conventional methods or some of the newer methods, such as RFLP analysis.

Since resistance to soybean looper in this study was determined to be additive, it should be possible to increase resistance in future cultivars by pyramiding additional genes from other sources of resistance. This can be done by conventional plant breeding techniques by utilizing soybean germplasm lines that show resistance to leaf-feeding insects and incorporating these genes into adapted cultivars or advanced breeding lines. The same goals could also be accomplished by any of the new methods of biotechnology that are currently available.

Additional research will need to be conducted on sources of resistance other than PI 229358-derived lines to determine how many other genes for resistance are available to breeders for utilization in their breeding programs. In order to fully exploit the benefits of insect resistance in a breeding program, it will become necessary to understand the mechanisms of resistance as well as the underlying genes that code for the mechanism. As new technology becomes available, the mysteries of the mechanisms of insect resistance will be solved. Ideally, the future promises the development of a resistant cultivar that has many genes for resistance that code for all three mechanisms of resistance.

APPENDIX A
LIST OF DEFOLIATION SCORES GENERATED BY WHOLE PLANT VISUAL,
PARTITIONED PLANT VISUAL, AND LEAF AREA OF THE PARTITIONED
PLANT RATING METHODS IN 1990.

List of defoliation scores generated by whole plant visual†, partitioned plant visual†, and leaf area of the partitioned plant‡ rating methods.

Observation	Plant	Whole Plant	Avg. Visual	Avg. Leaf Area
1	BBE-5-3	1	2.67	57.55
2	BBE-5-4	2	2.00	66.45
3	BBE-5-5	4	1.67	72.74
4	BBE-5-6	3	2.33	65.45
5	BBE-5-7	3	3.00	81.61
6	BBE-5-8	2	2.33	75.80
7	BBE-5-9	2	2.33	111.43
8	BBE-5-10	3	2.67	66.73
9	BBE-6-1	4	3.00	84.04
10	BBE-6-2	2	2.33	47.86
11	BBE-6-3	2	2.33	66.22
12	BBE-6-4	4	2.33	32.03
13	BBE-6-5	3	2.00	87.55
14	BBE-6-6	3	2.67	86.85
15	BBE-6-7	2	2.33	52.67
16	BBE-6-8	4	3.33	76.31
17	BBE-6-9	4	3.33	71.35
18	BBE-6-10	4	2.00	64.61
19	BBE-7-1	3	4.33	100.27
20	BBE-7-2	3	3.00	71.86
21	BBE-7-3	4	3.33	68.00
22	BBE-7-4	3	2.67	75.74
23	BBE-7-5	4	1.33	61.07
24	BBE-7-6	3	2.00	77.64
25	BBE-7-7	4	2.67	67.08
26	BBE-7-8	4	4.33	74.19
27	BBE-7-9	2	1.67	73.05
28	BBE-7-10	4	2.00	63.85
29	BBE-8-1	3	3.33	58.87
30	BBE-8-2	3	1.00	88.32
31	BBE-8-3	2	2.00	72.49
32	BBE-8-4	4	2.00	70.66
33	BBE-8-5	4	2.67	73.00
34	BBE-8-6	4	2.00	79.00

Observation	Plant	Whole Plant	Avg. Visual	Avg. Leaf Area
35	BBE-8-7	3	2.00	80.88
36	BBE-8-8	3	1.67	94.90
37	BBE-8-9	2	2.00	60.38
38	BBE-8-10	4	2.67	31.06
39	BBE-9-1	4	4.67	70.52
40	BBE-9-2	3	3.67	66.67
41	BBE-9-3	5	5.00	47.64
42	BBE-9-4	4	5.00	69.57
43	BBE-9-5	4	5.33	57.64
44	BBE-9-6	3	3.00	87.20
45	BBE-9-7	4	2.67	74.37
46	BBE-9-8	3	1.67	75.70
47	BBE-9-9	3	2.67	66.17
48	BBE-9-10	4	3.67	74.00
49	BBE-10-1	2	1.33	45.08
50	BBE-10-2	2	2.67	77.06
51	BBE-10-3	2	3.67	63.51
52	BBE-10-4	2	3.00	67.74
53	BBE-10-5	2	1.67	71.65
54	BBE-10-6	2	2.67	70.88
55	BBE-10-7	2	2.00	76.32
56	BBE-10-8	3	2.67	89.68
57	BBE-10-9	3	1.33	52.45
58	BBE-10-10	3	3.33	29.95
59	BBE-11-1	3	7.00	64.62
60	BBE-11-2	3	4.67	75.10
61	BBE-11-3	3	4.00	55.21
62	BBE-11-4	3	3.67	65.95
63	BBE-11-5	3	4.33	62.94
64	BBE-11-6	2	3.33	88.50
65	BBE-11-7	3	3.67	74.01
66	BBE-11-8	3	5.33	63.24
67	BBE-11-9	2	1.67	97.20
68	BBE-11-10	4	6.67	74.45
69	BBE-12-1	3	4.33	62.75
70	BBE-12-2	3	2.33	78.93

Observation	Plant	Whole Plant	Avg. Visual	Avg. Leaf Area
71	BBE-12-3	3	2.67	72.66
72	BBE-12-4	3	2.00	92.53
73	BBE-12-5	3	2.33	93.98
74	BBE-12-6	2	2.33	106.10
75	BBE-12-7	3	4.33	72.10
76	BBE-12-8	3	3.00	86.99
77	BBE-12-9	3	4.33	98.32
78	BBE-12-10	2	4.00	60.94
79	BBE-13-1	4	5.00	53.08
80	BBE-13-2	2	1.67	91.42
81	BBE-13-3	2	1.67	73.57
82	BBE-13-4	4	4.00	75.45
83	BBE-13-5	3	5.00	46.18
84	BBE-13-6	4	4.00	63.52
85	BBE-13-7	3	4.00	68.61
86	BBE-13-8	3	2.33	91.37
87	BBE-13-9	3	3.00	51.28
88	BBE-13-10	4	5.00	58.01
89	BBE-14-1	3	4.67	57.90
90	BBE-14-2	3	5.00	65.62
91	BBE-14-3	2	4.33	65.58
92	BBE-14-4	2	2.00	83.45
93	BBE-14-5	4	5.00	57.62
94	BBE-14-6	3	3.67	84.46
95	BBE-14-7	4	6.33	58.82
96	BBE-14-8	4	4.67	50.44
97	BBE-14-9	2	3.00	79.47
98	BBE-14-10	5	5.00	42.37
99	BBE-4-1	3	2.67	69.64
100	BBE-4-2	3	2.67	72.35
101	BBE-4-3	4	3.33	74.24
102	BBE-4-4	3	2.00	80.57
103	BBE-4-5	3	4.67	49.60
104	BBE-4-6	5	5.67	60.68
105	BBE-4-7	4	4.33	80.55
106	BBE-4-8	2	2.33	72.02

Observation	Plant	Whole Plant	Avg. Visual	Avg. Leaf Area
107	BBE-4-9	3	2.67	58.72
108	BBE-4-10	3	5.67	65.01
109	BBE-1-1	5	6.67	77.55
110	BBE-1-2	3	2.33	92.04
111	BBE-1-3	3	2.67	72.01
112	BBE-1-4	4	5.00	63.01
113	BBE-1-5	4	5.67	64.55
114	BBE-1-6	4	6.00	51.66
115	BBE-1-7	4	5.33	82.70
116	BBE-1-8	3	2.67	64.59
117	BBE-1-9	3	4.33	60.43
118	BBE-1-10	4	3.67	56.59
119	BBE-3-1	2	3.33	69.57
120	BBE-3-2	2	3.33	64.69
121	BBE-3-3	3	2.67	69.09
122	BBE-3-4	2	1.67	60.31
123	BBE-3-5	2	3.00	82.66
124	BBE-3-6	2	2.33	68.51
125	BBE-3-7	2	2.33	70.63
126	BBE-3-8	2	2.33	65.65
127	BBE-3-9	3	2.67	80.47
128	BBE-3-10	3	2.33	69.33
129	BBE-2-1	2	2.00	80.21
130	BBE-2-2	2	2.33	81.01
131	BBE-2-3	2	2.00	67.84
132	BBE-2-4	2	2.67	52.42
133	BBE-2-5	2	2.00	73.62
134	BBE-2-6	3	4.00	82.98
135	BBE-2-7	3	2.33	77.75
136	BBE-2-8	2	2.00	69.91
137	BBE-2-9	2	2.00	64.00
138	BBE-2-10	3	3.00	79.92
139	BBE-16-1	4	5.33	51.63
140	BBE-16-2	4	6.33	45.94
141	BBE-16-3	5	6.00	40.06
142	BBE-16-4	4	4.00	62.02

Observation	Plant	Whole Plant	Avg. Visual	Avg. Leaf Area
143	BBE-16-5	5	5.67	45.71
144	BBE-16-6	6	7.00	35.54
145	BBE-16-7	5	4.67	75.60
146	BBE-16-8	7	5.67	37.47
147	BBE-16-9	4	5.33	59.21
148	BBE-16-10	7	7.33	62.08
149	BBE-15-1	5	5.33	74.96
150	BBE-15-2	3	4.00	62.52
151	BBE-15-3	4	4.67	64.42
152	BBE-15-4	3	3.67	67.52
153	BBE-15-5	3	3.33	76.06
154	BBE-15-6	4	5.33	50.96
155	BBE-15-7	4	5.00	70.10
156	BBE-15-8	3	4.33	74.26
157	BBE-15-9	4	4.67	64.68
158	BBE-15-10	4	5.67	46.88
159	BBE-17-1	4	6.00	44.94
160	BBE-17-2	5	6.00	39.03
161	BBE-17-3	3	4.00	80.14
162	BBE-17-4	4	6.00	39.94
163	BBE-17-5	3	4.33	52.10
164	BBE-17-6	4	5.33	42.98
165	BBE-17-7	3	5.33	78.97
166	BBE-17-8	4	4.67	68.50
167	BBE-17-9	4	4.33	52.05
168	BBE-17-10	4	5.33	58.14
169	BBE-18-1	4	5.67	56.14
170	BBE-18-2	4	5.33	61.43
171	BBE-18-3	5	5.00	51.84
172	BBE-18-4	4	5.33	54.93
173	BBE-18-5	4	5.33	58.81
174	BBE-18-6	5	5.33	53.30
175	BBE-18-7	4	5.00	75.94
176	BBE-18-8	4	3.00	62.40
177	BBE-18-9	4	5.33	61.60
178	BBE-18-10	4	5.00	78.89

Observation	Plant	Whole Plant	Avg. Visual	Avg. Leaf Area
179	BBE-19-1	5	5.67	56.32
180	BBE-19-2	3	3.33	74.48
181	BBE-19-3	5	4.00	49.36
182	BBE-19-4	5	6.00	58.93
183	BBE-19-5	3	4.67	55.07
184	BBE-19-6	3	4.33	88.80
185	BBE-19-7	5	5.67	50.52
186	BBE-19-8	4	5.67	57.10
187	BBE-19-9	4	6.33	48.33
188	BBE-19-10	4	3.00	74.01
189	BBE-20-1	4	3.67	53.10
190	BBE-20-2	3	2.67	71.80
191	BBE-20-3	4	4.33	63.00
192	BBE-20-4	3	4.00	60.55
193	BBE-20-5	2	2.67	66.57
194	BBE-20-6	4	3.33	69.70
195	BBE-20-7	3	3.33	72.31
196	BBE-20-8	4	3.67	56.56
197	BBE-20-9	3	4.33	64.67
198	BBE-20-10	4	2.67	53.80
Mean (n=198)		3.32	3.68	67.13
Variance		0.98	2.07	201.92
Std.Dev.		0.99	1.44	14.21

† Based on a 1 to 10 scale divided into 10% increments with a 10 reflecting 91-100% defoliation.
‡ LI-COR LI-3000 portable leaf area meter measurements in cm^2 of leaf tissue.

APPENDIX B
LIST OF DEFOLIATION SCORES GENERATED BY WHOLE PLANT VISUAL,
PARTITIONED PLANT VISUAL, AND LEAF AREA OF THE PARTITIONED
PLANT RATING METHODS IN 1991.

List of defoliation scores† generated by whole plant visual, partitioned plant visual, and leaf area of the partitioned plant‡ rating methods.

Observation	Cage	Plant	Whole plant	Avg. visual	Avg. LICOR
1	1	9	3	2.00	1.67
2	1	197	5	4.00	2.00
3	1	214	4	3.00	3.00
4	1	15	8	7.00	5.00
5	1	250	-§	-	-
6	1	235	4	4.33	2.00
7	1	63	6	6.67	5.00
8	1	180	2	2.00	1.33
9	1	61	3	3.33	2.67
10	1	42	4	3.67	2.00
11	1	223	3	3.67	4.00
12	1	150	6	5.00	4.00
13	1	186	8	7.67	5.00
14	1	26	2	3.00	2.33
15	1	225	3	2.67	2.33
16	1	187	7	5.67	4.67
17	1	3	2	3.33	1.33
18	1	248	8	6.67	6.33
19	1	17	9	7.67	7.00
20	1	196	8	8.00	6.00
21	1	222	4	3.67	3.00
22	1	275	5	7.00	5.00
23	1	8	2	3.67	1.67
24	1	158	7	5.67	4.33
25	1	166	7	7.67	4.00
26	1	140	8	8.00	5.67
27	1	141	4	5.33	2.33
28	1	138	2	3.67	2.33
29	1	85	5	5.00	3.33
30	1	244	4	4.33	3.00
31	1	122	3	5.33	2.00
32	1	144	8	8.33	6.00
33	1	105	5	5.33	3.00
34	1	92	6	6.67	4.67
35	1	126	8	8.33	6.00
36	1	67	7	7.00	5.00
37	1	51	6	8.67	6.00
38	1	75	7	8.33	4.67
39	1	80	5	6.33	3.33

Observation	Cage	Plant	Whole plant	Avg. visual	Avg. LICOR
40	1	178	4	5.33	3.33
41	1	179	5	6.00	4.00
42	1	22	8	7.67	4.67
43	1	110	7	6.33	5.00
44	1	270	9	8.67	7.00
45	1	212	-	-	-
46	1	100	6	5.67	2.67
47	1	213	3	4.33	2.00
48	1	25	2	4.00	3.00
49	1	103	5	5.67	2.67
50	1	79	3	3.67	3.00
51	2	248	4	3.33	1.67
52	2	213	2	3.33	3.33
53	2	17	8	8.33	5.67
54	2	270	8	9.00	4.33
55	2	150	5	5.67	4.00
56	2	100	4	5.00	3.00
57	2	194	6	6.67	3.33
58	2	186	6	5.67	4.00
59	2	61	7	7.67	5.00
60	2	79	4	4.00	2.67
61	2	9	4	3.00	4.33
62	2	250	9	9.33	6.33
63	2	26	2	2.33	1.67
64	2	222	7	6.00	5.00
65	2	214	1	3.33	2.00
66	2	244	2	4.00	2.00
67	2	103	5	6.33	3.00
68	2	178	3	4.67	3.00
69	2	22	8	8.67	5.33
70	2	85	7	5.33	5.33
71	2	180	3	5.00	2.67
72	2	42	3	6.33	5.00
73	2	110	5	4.67	3.33
74	2	212	-	-	-
75	2	275	5	5.00	3.33
76	2	158	6	7.00	3.00
77	2	51	4	4.33	3.00
78	2	75	5	6.33	3.33
79	2	25	5	2.00	1.67
80	2	8	3	3.00	1.67

Observation	Cage	Plant	Whole plant	Avg. visual	Avg. LICOR
81	2	140	8	4.67	2.33
82	2	15	3	8.67	5.00
83	2	138	3	2.67	1.33
84	2	67	6	6.67	3.33
85	2	126	7	8.00	6.00
86	2	63	8	7.67	5.33
87	2	179	6	7.33	5.33
88	2	80	7	7.67	2.67
89	2	92	6	6.67	2.00
90	2	3	3	4.33	2.00
91	2	223	4	6.67	3.33
92	2	166	5	7.00	4.00
93	2	122	2	3.67	2.33
94	2	225	3	4.67	2.00
95	2	196	9	9.00	5.33
96	2	144	9	9.00	5.00
97	2	187	3	5.33	2.33
98	2	105	4	6.33	3.00
99	2	141	3	4.33	3.00
100	2	235	5	7.67	3.00
Mean (N=97)			5.10	5.65	3.62
Variance			4.70	3.88	2.19
Std.Dev.			2.17	1.97	1.48

† Based on a 1 to 10 scale divided into 10% increments with a 10 reflecting 91-100% defoliation.
‡ Based on LI-COR LI-3000 portable leaf area meter measurements that have been converted to % defoliation and categorized into the 1-to-10 scale.
§ Missing data points.

APPENDIX C
GENERATION MEANS ANALYSIS
SAS PROGRAM

```
OPTIONS LS=80 PS=60;
/*This is a Generation Means Analysis based on Hayman's methodology, Heredity
12:371-390 */
DATA;
INFILE 'A:Cage1.dat';
/* The INPUT statement will vary according to the data set, you need generation
("GEN") and a dependent variable */
INPUT row plant gen $ fc$ rating1 rating2 rating3;
MEANRATE = (rating1+rating2+rating3)/3;
PROC SORT; BY GEN;
PROC MEANS; BY GEN; VAR MEANRATE;
OUTPUT OUT=NE MEAN=Y VAR=V STDERR=S;
DATA NEW; SET NE; RS=1/S; IF GEN='D' OR GEN='BD' THEN DELETE;
PROC PRINT;
/* You need a minimum of 6 generations to conduct this analysis, if the number of
generations used are different than the amount (9) in this example, refer to Gamble's
paper (Canadian J. Plant Sci. 42:339-348) to obtain the proper coefficients. Another
source of information is Jennings, et al. (IA State J. Research, 48:267-280) */
DATA COEFCNTS;

        INPUT GEN $ X1 X2 X3 X4 X5;
        CARDS;
        BC1  0.5  0.0  0.25  0.0  0.0
        BC2 -0.5  0.0  0.25  0.0  0.0
        BS1  0.5 -0.25 0.25 -0.25 0.0625
        BS2 -0.5 -0.25 0.25  0.25 0.0625
        F1   0.0  0.5  0.0   0.0  0.25
        F2   0.0  0.0  0.0   0.0  0.0
        F3   0.0 -0.25 0.0   0.0  0.0625
        P1   1.0 -0.5  1.0  -1.0  0.25
        P2  -1.0 -0.5  1.0   1.0  0.25

DATA FINAL; MERGE NEW COEFCNTS;
PROC PRINT;
```

```
/* This model tests the significance of the additive (X1) and the dominant (X2) effects
*/
TITLE 'PROC REG WEIGHTED';
PROC REG;
MODEL Y = X1 X2;
WEIGHT RS;
/* The model must be weighted to account for the unequal population sizes among the
generations. See Rowe and Alexander, Crop Sci. 20:109-110, for further detail. The next
model tests for the epistatic effects, additive-additive (X3), additive-dominant (X4), and
dominant-dominant (X5), as well as the additive (X1) and dominant (X2) effects. */
PRO REG;
MODEL Y = X1 X2 X3 X4 X5;
WEIGHT RS;
RUN;

/* This next set of models are tested with PROC GLM instead of PROC REG */
TITLE 'PROC GLM WEIGHTED';
PROC GLM;
MODEL Y = X1 X2;
WEIGHT RS;
PROC GLM;
MODEL Y = X1 X2 X3 X4 X5;
WEIGHT RS;
RUN;

/* The next series of models are the same as the previous models, except that they
assume equal population size among the generations, and are therefore not weighted. */
TITLE 'PROC REG NOWEIGHT';
PROC REG;
MODEL Y = X1 X2;
PROC REG;
MODEL Y = X1 X2 X3 X4 X5;
RUN;
TITLE 'PROC GLM NOWEIGHT';
MODEL Y = X1 X2;
PROC GLM;
MODEL Y = X1 X2 X3 X4 X5;
RUN;
/* Depending on whether or not the population sizes among the generations are equal,
report the model that has the most significant effects from either PROC GLM or PROC
REG. */
```

GENERATION MEANS ANALYSIS
SAS PROGRAM

```
/* This is a Generation Means Analysis that is based on Hayman's methodology,
Heredity 12:371-390.  This analysis tests for block effects as well as estimating the
additive, dominant, and epistatic effects. */
DATA A;
INFILE 'A:CAGE1.DAT';CAGE=1;
/* The INPUT statement will vary according to the data set, you need generation
("GEN") and a dependent variable. */
INPUT ROW PLANT GEN $ FC $ RATING1 RATING2 RATING3;
MEANRATE = (RATING1+RATING2+RATING3)/3;
DATA B;
INFILE 'A:CAGE2.DAT';CAGE=2;
INPUT ROW PLANT GEN $ FC $ RATING1 RATING2 RATING3;
MEANRATE = (RATING1+RATING2+RATING3)/3;
DATA BOTH;SET A B;RUN;
PROC SORT; BY CAGE GEN;
PROC MEANS; BY CAGE GEN; VAR MEANRATE;
OUTPUT OUT=NE MEAN=Y VAR=V STDERR=S;
DATA NEW; SET NE; RS=1/S;IF GEN='D'OR GEN='BD' THEN DELETE; PROC
PRINT;
/* You need a minimum of 6 generations to conduct this analysis, if the number of
generations used are different than the amount (9) in this example, refer to Gamble's
paper (Canadian J. Plant Sci. 42:339-348) to obtain the proper coefficients. Another
source of information is Jennings, et al. (IA State J. Research, 48:267-280) */
DATA COEFCNTS;

  INPUT CAGE GEN $ X1 X2 X3 X4 X5;
  CARDS;
1   BC1  0.5  0.0  0.25  0.0  0.0
1   BC2 -0.5  0.0  0.25  0.0  0.0
1   BS1  0.5 -0.25 0.25 -0.25 0.0625
1   BS2 -0.5 -0.25 0.25  0.25 0.0625
1   F1   0.0  0.5  0.0   0.0  0.25
1   F2   0.0  0.0  0.0   0.0  0.0
1   F3   0.0 -0.25 0.0   0.0  0.0625
```

```
1  P1    1.0 -0.5  1.0  -1.0  0.25
1  P2   -1.0 -0.5  1.0   1.0  0.25
2  BC1   0.5  0.0  0.25  0.0  0.0
2  BC2  -0.5  0.0  0.25  0.0  0.0
2  BS1   0.5 -0.25 0.25 -0.25 0.0625
2  BS2  -0.5 -0.25 0.25  0.25 0.0625
2  F1    0.0  0.5  0.0   0.0  0.25
2  F2    0.0  0.0  0.0   0.0  0.0
2  F3    0.0 -0.25 0.0   0.0  0.0625
2  P1    1.0 -0.5  1.0  -1.0  0.25
2  P2   -1.0 -0.5  1.0   1.0  0.25


PROC SORT DATA=COEFCNTS;BY CAGE GEN;
DATA FINAL; MERGE NEW COEFCNTS;BY CAGE GEN;
PROC PRINT;
/* This model tests the significance of the additive (X1) and dominant (X2) effects */
PROC GLM DATA=FINAL;BY CAGE;
MODEL Y = X1 X2 /SS1 SS3;
WEIGHT RS;
/* The model must be weighted to account for the unequal population sizes among the
generations. See Rowe and Alexander, Crop Sci. 20:109-110, for further detail. */
PROC GLM DATA=FINAL;CLASS CAGE;
MODEL Y = CAGE X1 X2 CAGE*X1 CAGE*X2/SS1 SS3 SOLUTION;
WEIGHT RS;
PROC GLM DATA=FINAL;CLASS CAGE;
MODEL Y = CAGE X1 X2 /SS1 SS3 SOLUTION;
WEIGHT RS;
/* The next model tests for the epistatic effects, additive-additive (X3), additive-dominant
(X4), and dominant-dominant (X5), as well as the additive (X1) and dominant (X2)
effects. */
PROC GLM;BY CAGE;
MODEL Y = X1 X2 X3 X4 X5;
WEIGHT RS;
RUN;
PROC GLM;CLASS CAGE;
MODEL Y = CAGE X1 X2 X3 X4 X5 CAGE*X1 CAGE*X2 CAGE*X3 CAGE*X4
CAGE*X5/SS1 SS3 SOLUTION;
WEIGHT RS;
RUN;
PROC GLM;CLASS CAGE;
MODEL y = CAGE X1 X2 X3 X4 X5 /SS1 SS3 SOLUTION;
WEIGHT RS;
RUN;
```

$$\bar{x} = [1(0.5) + 33(1.5) + 78(2.5) + 154(3.5) + 39(4.5) + 6(5.5) + 2(6.5) + 1(7.5)]/314$$
$$= 3.2$$

$$s^2 = [1(0.5-3.2)^2 + 33(1.5-3.2)^2 + 78(2.5-3.2)^2 + 159(3.5-3.2)^2 + 39(4.5-3.2)^2 + 6(5.5-3.2)^2 + 2(6.5-3.2)^2 + 1(7.5-3.2)^2]/(314-1)$$
$$= 0.9343$$

$$s = (0.9343)^{\frac{1}{2}}$$
$$= 0.96662$$

Next, the value x was calculated for each class as follows:

Class 1	$x = (3.2 - 0.5)/0.96662 = 2.30701$
Class 2	$x = (3.2 - 1.5)/0.96662 = 1.27248$
Class 3	$x = (3.2 - 2.5)/0.96662 = 0.23794$
Class 4	$x = (3.2 - 3.5)/0.96662 = -0.79659$
Class 5	$x = (3.2 - 4.5)/0.96662 = -1.83112$
Class 6	$x = (3.2 - 5.5)/0.96662 = -2.86566$
Class 7	$x = (3.2 - 6.5)/0.96662 = -3.90019$
Class 8	$x = (3.2 - 7.5)/0.96662 = -4.93472$

The corresponding Z value for each class was obtained by finding x in a table of probabilities of the normal distribution (76). The Z value obtained for each class was then subtracted from one and multiplied by 100% to obtain the theoretical % of the population that fell into each class. The theoretical number of each class was obtained by multiplying the total n of the population by the theoretical % of each class. This was done for each class as shown below:

x	Z	1.000 - Z	Theoretical % Class	Theoretical Distribution
2.30701	0.99111	0.00889	0.89	3
1.27248	0.89796	0.10204	9.32	29
0.23794	0.59484	0.40516	30.31	95
-0.79659	0.21185	0.78815	38.30	120
-1.83112	0.03362	0.96638	17.82	56
-2.86566	0.00205	0.99795	3.16	10
-3.90019	0.00005	0.99995	0.2	1
-4.93472	0.00001	0.99999	0.004	0

The observed versus theoretical distribution of the F_2 population was then tested with a X^2 test.

REFERENCES

1. Allard, R.W. 1960. Principles of plant breeding. John Wiley and Sons, Inc. New York, NY.

2. Anonymous. 1979. USDA agricultural statistics. U.S. Gov. Print. Office, Washington, D.C.

3. Anonymous. 1990. USDA agricultural statistics. U.S. Gov. Print. Office, Washington, D.C.

4. Berger, R.D. 1988. Measuring disease intensity. p.1-4. *In* Biological and cultural tests for control of plant diseases. American Phytopathological Society Press, St. Paul, MN.

5. Bowers, G.R. 1990. Registration of 'Crockett' soybean. Crop Sci. 30:427.

6. Briggs, F.N., and P.F. Knowles. 1967. Introduction to plant breeding. Reinhold Publishing Corporation, .

7. Campbell, C.L., and L.V. Madden. 1990. Introduction to plant disease epidemiology. John Wiley and Sons, New York, NY.

8. Chapman, S.R., and F.H. McNeal. 1970. Gene effects for protein in five spring wheat crosses. Crop Sci. 10:45-46.

9. Chiang, H.S., D.M. Norris, A. Ciepiela, A. Oosterwyk, P. Shapiro, and M. Jackson. 1986. Comparitive constitutive resistance in soybean lines to Mexican bean beetle. Entomol. Exp. Appl. 42:19-26.

10. Chiu, P. S-B., and M.H. Bass. 1978. Soybean looper: susceptibility of larvae to insecticides. J. Ga. Entomol. Soc. 13:169-173.

11. Cooper, R.L., and R.B. Hammond. 1988. Registration of Mexican bean beetle resistant germplasm line HC83-1239. Crop Sci. 28:1037-1038.

12. Deren, C.W., and K.H. Quesenberry. 1989. Inheritance of photoperiod-induced flowering in three photoperiodic lines of *Aeschynomene americana* L. Theor. Appl. Genet. 78:825-830.

13. Diers, B.W., L. Mansur, J. Imsande, and R.C. Shoemaker. 1992. Mapping phytophthora resistance loci in soybean with restriction fragment length polymorphism markers. Crop Sci. 32:377-383.

14. Ennis, W.B., Jr. 1976. Modern methods for controlling pests. p. 375-386. *In* L.D. Hill (ed.) World soybean research. Interstate Printers and Publishers. Danville, IL.

15. Entomological Society of America, Southeastern Branch, Insect Detection, Evaluation, and Predication Committee. 1984. Insect detection, evaluation and prediction report [for] 1982, v.7. MS State, MS.

16. Entomological Society of America, Southeastern Branch, Insect Detection, Evaluation, and Predication Committee. 1985. Insect detection, evaluation and prediction report [for] 1984, v.9. Clemson, SC.

17. Fehr, W.R., and C.E. Caviness. 1977. Stages of soybean development. Agric. and Home Economics Exp. Stn. and Cooperative Ext. Serv., Iowa State Univ. and Arkansas Agric. Exp. Stn. Spec. Rep. 80.

18. Felland, C.M., H.N. Pitre, R.G. Luttrell, and J.L. Hamer. 1990. Resistance to pyrethroid insecticides in soybean looper (Lepidoptera:Noctuidae) in Mississippi. J. Econ. Entomol. 83:35-40.

19. Funderburk, J.E., A.R. Soffes, R.D. Barnett, D.C. Herzog, and K. Hinson. 1990. Plot size and shape in relation to soybean resistance for velvetbean caterpillar (Lepidoptera:Noctuidae). J. Econ. Entomol. 83:2107-2110.

20. Funderburk, J.E., D.L. Wright, and I.D. Teare. 1990. Preplant tillage effects on population dynamics of soybean insect pests. Crop Sci. 30:686-690.

21. Gamble, E.E. 1962. Gene effects in corn (*Zea mays* L.) I.separation and relative importance of gene effects for yield. Canadian J. Plant Sci. 42:339-348.

22. Gary, D.J., L. Lambert, and J.D. Ouzts. 1985. Evaluation of soybean plant introductions for resistance to foliar feeding insects. J. MS Academy Sci. 30:67-82.

23. Hallauer, A.R., and J.B. Miranda. 1981. Quantitative genetics in maize breeding. Iowa State Univ. Press, Ames, IA.

24. Hamer, J.L. 1990. Soybean looper: biology and approaches for improved management. Mississippi Cooperative Extension Service Information Sheet 1400.

25. Hart, S.V., J.W. Burton, and W.V. Campbell. 1988. Comparison of three techniques to evaluate advanced breeding lines of soybean for leaf-feeding resistance to corn earworm (Lepidoptera:Noctuidae). J. Econ Entomol. 81:615-620.

26. Hartley, G.G. 1990. Multicellular rearing methods for the beet armyworm, soybean looper, and velvetbean caterpillar (Lepidoptera:Noctuidae). J. Entomol. Sci. 25:336-340.

27. Hartwig, E.E., and J.M. Epps. 1967. Registration of Centennial soybeans. Crop Sci. 17:979.

28. Hartwig, E.E., L. Lambert, and T.C. Kilen. 1990. Registration of Lamar soybean. Crop Sci. 30:231.

29. Hartwig, E.E., S.G. Turnipseed, and T.C. Kilen. 1984. Registration of soybean germplasm line D75-10169. Crop Sci. 24:214-215.

30. Hatchett, J.H., G.L. Beland, and T.C. Kilen. 1979. Identification of multiple insect resistant soybean lines. Crop Sci. 19:557-559.

31. Hayman, B.I. 1958. The separation of epistatic from additive and dominance variation in generation means. Heredity 12:371-390.

32. Hinson, K., R.A. Kinlock, H.A. Peacock, W.H. Chapman, and W.T. Scudder. 1981. Braxton soybean. Florida Agric. Exp. Stn. Circular S-276.

33. Horsfall, J.G., and R.W. Barratt. 1945. An improved grading system for measuring plant disease. Phytopathology 35:655(abstr.).

34. Jennings, C.W., W.A. Russell, W.D. Guthrie, and R.L. Grindeland. 1974. Genetics of resistance in maize to second-brood European corn borer. Iowa State J. Research 48:267-280.

35. Joshi, J.M., and M. Nobakht. 1988. Evaluation of commercial soybean cultivars and advance breeding lines for nonpreference to *Heliothis zea*. Soybean Genetics Newsletter. 15:124-126.

36. Kilen, T.C., J.H. Hatchett, and E.E. Hartwig. 1977. Evaluation of early generation soybeans for resistance to soybean looper. Crop Sci. 17:397-398.

37. Kilen, T.C., and L. Lambert. 1986. Evidence for different genes controlling insect resistance in three soybean genotypes. Crop Sci. 26:869-871.

38. Kogan, M. 1982. Plant resistance in pest management. p. 93-134. *In* R.L. Metcalf and W.H. Luckmann (ed.) Introduction to insect pest management. 2nd ed. John Wiley and Sons, New York, NY.

39. Kogan, M. 1986. Natural chemicals in plant resistance to insects. Iowa State J. Research 60:501-527.

40. Kogan, M., and D.E. Kuhlman. 1982. Soybean insects: identification and management in Illinois. Illinois Agric. Exp. Stn. Bull. 773.

41. Kogan, M., and S.G. Turnipseed. 1980. Soybean growth and assessment of damage by arthropods. p.3-29. *In* M. Kogan and D.C. Herzog (eds.) Sampling methods in soybean entomology. Springer, New York, NY.

42. Kraemer, M.E., M. Rangappa, P.S. Benepal, and T. Mebrahtu. 1988. Field evaluation of soybeans for Mexican bean beetle resistance. I. Maturity groups VI, VII, and VIII. Crop Sci. 28:497-499.

43. Lambert, L. 1984. An improved screen-cage design for use in plant and insect research. Agron. J. 76:168-170.

44. Lambert, L., and J.L. Hamer. 1988. Evaluation of 10 soybean cultivars for relative levels of damage by two insect species. Mississippi Agric. and Forestry Expt. Stn. Res. Rep. 13(5).

45. Lambert, L., and T.C. Kilen. 1984a. Influence of three soybean plant genotypes and their F_1 intercrosses on the development of five insect species. J. Econ. Entomol. 77:622-625.

46. Lambert, L., and T.C. Kilen. 1984b. Insect resistance factor in soybean PI's 229358 and 227687 demonstrated by grafting. Crop Sci. 24:163-165.

47. Lambert, L., and T.C. Kilen. 1984c. Multiple insect resistance in several soybean genotypes. Crop Sci. 24:887-890.

48. Leonard, B.R., D.J. Boethel, A.N. Sparks, Jr., M.B. Layton, J.S. Mink, A.M. Pavloff, E. Burris, and J.B. Graves. 1990. Variations in response of soybean looper (Lepidoptera: Noctuidae) to selected insecticides in Louisiana. J. Econ. Entomol. 83:27-34.

49. Leonard, W.H., H.O. Mann, and L. Powers. 1957. Partitioning method of genetic analysis applied to plant-height inheritance in barley. Colo. Agric. Exp. Stn. Tech. Bull. 60:2-24.

50. Luckmann, W.H., and R.L. Metcalf. 1982. The pest management concept. p. 1-28. *In* R.L. Metcalf and W.H. Luckmann (ed.) Introduction to insect pest management. 2nd ed. John Wiley and Sons, New York, NY.

51. Mather, K., and J.L. Jinks. 1971. Biometrical genetics. 2nd ed. Chapman and Hall, London.

52. McKenna, T., L. Lambert, J.D. Ouzts, and T.C. Kilen. 1988. Evaluation of wild soybean, *Glycine soja*, for resistance to foliar feeding insects. J. MS Academy Sci. 33:17-24.

53. Mebrahtu, T., W.J. Kenworthy, and T.C. Elden. 1988. Inorganic nutrient analysis of leaf tissue from soybean lines screened for Mexican bean beetle resistance. J. Entomol. Sci. 23:44-51.

54. Mebrahtu, T., W.J. Kenworthy, and T.C. Elden. 1990. Genetic study of resistance to the Mexican bean beetle in soybean lines. J. Genect. and Breed. 44:7-12.

55. Meredith, W.R., Jr., and R.R. Bridge. 1972. Heterosis and gene action in cotton, *Gossypium hirsutum* L. Crop Sci. 12:304-310.

56. Meredith, W.R., and M.L. Laster. 1975. Agronomic and genetic analysis of tarnished plant bug tolerance in cotton. Crop Sci. 15:535-538.

57. Painter, R.H. 1968. Insect resistance in crop plants. The Univ. Press of Kansas, Lawerence, KS.

58. Pedigo, L.P. 1989. Entomology and pest management. Macmillan, New York, NY.

59. Plaut, J.L., and R.D. Berger. 1980. Development of *Cercosporidium personatum* in three peanut canopy layers. Peanut Sci. 7:46-49.

60. Poehlman, J.M. 1987. Breeding field crops. 3rd ed. Van Nostrand Reinhold, New York, NY.

61. Powers, L., and L.F. Locke. 1950. Partitioning method of genetic analysis applied to quantitative characters of tomato crosses. USDA Tech. Bull. No. 998.

62. Rose, R.L., B.R. Leonard, T.C. Sparks, and J.B. Graves. 1990. Enhanced metabolism and knockdown resistance in a field versus a laboratory strain of the soybean looper (Lepidoptera: Noctuidae). J. Econ. Entomol. 83:672-677.

63. Rose, R.L., T.C. Sparks, and C.M. Smith. 1989. The influence of resistant soybean (PI 227687) foliage and coumestrol on the metabolism of xenobiotics by the soybean looper, *Pseudoplusia includens* (Walker). Pest. Biochem. and Physiol. 34:17-26.

64. Rowan, G.B., H.R. Boerma, J.N. All, and J. Todd. 1991. Soybean cultivar resistance to defoliating insects. Crop Sci. 31:678-682.

65. Rowe, K.E., and W.L. Alexander. 1980. Computations for estimating the genetic parameters in joint-scaling tests. Crop Sci. 20:109-110.

66. Ruesink, W.G. 1980. Introduction to sampling theory. p 61-77. *In* M. Kogan and D.C.Herzog (eds.) Sampling methods in soybean methodology. Springer, New York, NY.

67. Sage, G.M.C., and M.J. de Isturiz. 1974. The inheritance of anther extrusion in two spring wheat varieties. Theor. Appl. Genet. 45:126-133.

68. SAS Institute. 1990. SAS/STAT user's guide. Vols. 1 and 2. SAS Inst., Inc., Cary, NC.

69. Schillinger, J.A. 1976. Host plant resistance to insects in soybeans. p.579-583. *In* L.D. Hill (ed.) World soybean research. Interstate Printers and Publishers. Danville, IL.

70. Scott, G.E., A.R. Hallauer, and F.F. Dicke. 1964. Types of gene action conditioning resistance to European corn borer leaf feeding. Crop Sci. 4:603-605.

71. Shokes, F.M., R.D. Berger, D.H. Smith, and J.M. Rasp. 1987. Reliability of disease assessment procedures: a case study with late leafspot of peanut. Oleagineux 42:245-251.

72. Sisson, V.A., P.A. Miller, W.V. Campbell, and J.W. Van Duyn. 1976. Evidence of inheritance of resistance to the Mexican bean beetle in soybeans. Crop Sci. 16:835-837.

73. Smith, C.M. 1985. Expression, mechanisms, and chemistry of resistance in soybean, *Glycine max* L. (Merr.) to the soybean looper, *Psuedoplusia includens* (Walker). Insect Sci. Applic. 6:243-248.

74. Smith, C.M. 1989.Plant resistance to insects: a fundamental approach. John Wiley and Sons, New York, NY.

75. Smith, K.J., and W. Huyser. 1987. World distribution and significance of soybean. *In* J.R. Wilcox (ed.) Soybean: improvement, production, and uses. 2nd ed. Agronomy 16:1-22.

76. Snedecor, G.W., and W.G. Cochran. 1989. Statistical methods. 8th. ed. Iowa State University Press, Ames, IA.

77. Sokal, R.F., and F.J. Rohlf. 1981. Biometry. 2nd. ed. W.H. Freeman and Company, New York, NY.

78. Southwood, T.R.E. 1978. Ecological methods with particular reference to the study of insect populations. 2nd. ed. Chapman and Hall, New York, NY.

79. Sullivan, M.J. 1985. Resistance to insect defoliators. *In* R. Shibles (ed.) World Research Conference III: Proceedings. Westview Press, Boulder, CO.

80. Talekar, N.S., H.R. Lee, and Suharsono. 1988. Resistance of soybean to four defoliator species in Taiwan. J. Econ. Entomol. 81:1469-1473.

81. Tester, C.F. 1977. Constituents of soybean cultivars differing in insect resistance. Phytochemistry. 16:1899-1901.

82. Turnipseed, S.G., and M.J. Sullivan. 1976. Plant resistance in soybean insect management. p.549-560. *In* L.D. Hill (ed.) World Soybean Research. Interstate Printers and Publishers. Danville, IL.

83. Van Duyn, J.W., S.G. Turnipseed, and J.D. Maxwell. 1971. Resistance in soybeans to the Mexican bean beetle: I. Sources of resistance. Crop Sci. 11:572-573.

BIOGRAPHICAL SKETCH

Michael Montgomery Kenty was born on August 27, 1959 in San Antonio, Texas. He completed his secondary education at Greenville High School, Greenville, Mississippi in 1977. In 1977, he initiated his undergraduate studies at the University of Mississippi in Botany. He received a Bachelor of Science in Agronomy at Mississippi State University in 1983.

Prior to graduation he joined the staff of Sandoz Crop Protection Research, where he conducted pesticide evaluations until September, 1986. In December, 1986, he joined the staff of the USDA-ARS Soybean Production Research Unit at Stoneville, Mississippi as an Agronomist. In December, 1988, he was awarded a Masters of Science in Natural Science from Delta State University. In September, 1989, he took a leave of absence from the USDA and entered the University of Florida. Currently, he is a candidate for the degree of Doctor of Philosophy, Department of Agronomy, University of Florida.

I certify that I have read this study and that in my opinion it conforms to acceptable standards of scholarly presentation and is fully adequate, in scope and quality, as a dissertation for the degree of Doctor of Philosophy.

Kuell Hinson, Chair
Professor of Agronomy

I certify that I have read this study and that in my opinion it conforms to acceptable standards of scholarly presentation and is fully adequate, in scope and quality, as a dissertation for the degree of Doctor of Philosophy.

Kenneth H. Quesenberry
Professor of Agronomy

I certify that I have read this study and that in my opinion it conforms to acceptable standards of scholarly presentation and is fully adequate, in scope and quality, as a dissertation for the degree of Doctor of Philosophy.

David S. Wofford
Associate Professor of Agronomy

I certify that I have read this study and that in my opinion it conforms to acceptable standards of scholarly presentation and is fully adequate, in scope and quality, as a dissertation for the degree of Doctor of Philosophy.

John R. Strayer
Professor of Entomology and Nematology

I certify that I have read this study and that in my opinion it conforms to acceptable standards of scholarly presentation and is fully adequate, in scope and quality, as a dissertation for the degree of Doctor of Philosophy.

Joseph E. Funderburk
Associate Professor of
Entomology and Nematology

This dissertation was submitted to the Graduate Faculty of the College of Agriculture and to the Graduate School and was accepted as partial fulfillment of the requirements for the degree of Doctor of Philosophy.

April 1994

Jack L. Fry

_____
Dean, College of Agriculture

_____
Dean, Graduate School

CPSIA information can be obtained
at www.ICGtesting.com
Printed in the USA
BVHW011659100619

550610BV00011B/515/P